D0380867

PUT HEMORRHOIDS AND CONSTIPATION BEHIND YOU

Kenneth Yasny, Ph.D.

East Canaan, Connecticut
Safe Goods Publishing

© Copyright 1997 by Kenneth Yasny

ISBN #1884820220
Library of Congress #96-070945

Publisher: Safe Goods Publishing
                    PO Box 36
                    East Canaan, CT 06024

All rights reserved. This book may not be duplicated in any way without the expressed written consent of the publisher, except in the form of brief excerpts or quotations for the purposes of review. The information contained herein is for the personal use of the reader and may not be incorporated in any commercial programs, other books, without prior written permission of the publisher or author.

Table of Contents

Dedication

This book is dedicated to my dad,
who inspired me to be the best person I can be.

And to all those who have suffered
with digestive problems.

CAUTION

The information presented in this book is not intended as a diagnosis of health problems or as a replacement for professional medical care.

If you have a specific health problem or if you have further questions, please consult your local health professional. The instructions and advice contained in this book is in no way intended as a substitute for medical counseling.

QUANTITY DISCOUNTS are available to **Schools, Corporations, and Professional Organizations** who would like to use this book for training, fund raising, and other educational purposes.

For information, contact:
Safe Goods Publishing
PO Box 36
E. Canaan, CT 06024

Tel: 860-824-5302
Fax: 941-484-5951
e-mail: safe@snet.net

Acknowledgments

Without the help of the following people, I could not have written this book: Sam Friedman, my "partner in health," worked in the background to set up *The Colon Health Society*. Without Sam, this book would never have found its way to so many people. Jamie, my partner, inspired me to continue when I had seemingly lost all energy. Arlette, my sister, first exposed me to the ideas of natural health that tempted me away from the field of traditional medicine. My mother, who gave of her time unstintingly, read my work and gave invaluable advice. Fox, who edited my notes, turned them into a smoothly running river of coherent thought. Laka gave me her keen insights and her energy, even when she needed energy herself. Sarah Toll for making our book look so pretty. Jim O'Connor breathed vigor into all of us involved with this project at those times when we were most exhausted. To Lori on flow control, and to Jason for his design wisdom. And, finally, I'd like to thank our sponsors, who contributed to making this project happen.

Companion Workbook - Now Available

Due to numerous requests, we've developed a companion workbook for *Put Hemorrhoids & Constipation Behind You.*

Although the book and workbook are each valuable on their own, taking advantage of both will greatly facilitate the learning and healing process. While the book provides background information, theoretical discussion, and thorough explanation, the workbook is a detailed road map that guides you through a step-by-step approach to healing hemorrhoids and constipation.

Specifically, the workbook will allow you to:

- Evaluate your specific situation.
- Design a healing program tailored to your exact needs.
- Work through a step-by-step regimen that will help you eliminate hemorrhoids and constipation.
- Improve your general health and prevent future colon problems.

For information regarding *Put Hemorrhoids & Constipation Behind You, The Colon Health Workbook, "The Colon Health Video,"* or boxed sets, please contact:

The Colon Health Society
505 S. Beverly Drive #438
Beverly Hills, CA 90212
Tel: 800-745-0791
Fax: 310-277-8952
www.colonhealth.com
esteem@starone.com

Introduction

By Sam Friedman

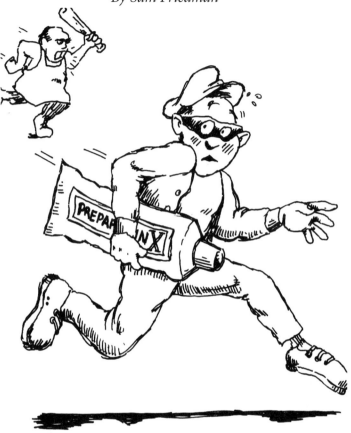

Life sometimes takes us in directions we never dreamed of, and here I am writing an introduction to a book on a topic that makes me a bit uneasy. Like most people, I'd rather not discuss hemorrhoids and constipation; quite frankly, I wish I could avoid the subject altogether.

As with most good health books, this one evolved from personal experience. I think most of us tend to get involved in health issues either because we have an experience that affects us personally in some profound way or because the light goes on and we see a problem that needs to be explored, perhaps for the benefit of everyone.

Both of these hold true for me. Having suffered from both hemorrhoids and constipation for many years, this subject hits close to home. The idea of creating a resource to help people put hemorrhoids and constipation behind them seemed like a wonderful thing to do, especially since both these problems are preventable.

Everyone I spoke with thought this was a great idea. "Why didn't somebody think of this before?" some wondered. Others asked "How soon can I get a copy?" or told me, "I've been looking for this for a long time."

Hemorrhoids afflict more than half of us at some point in our lives, and constipation, which is often associated with hemorrhoids, affects an even greater number than that. Strangely though, few people can even spell the word hemorrhoid and almost everyone is too embarrassed to even talk about the problem. I was rather shocked to find out that the second most common item lifted from drug stores and pharmacies is Preparation H™. It isn't that people can't afford the few dollars it costs, but rather, they are just too embarrassed to walk up to the cashier and admit that they have this "dreaded" problem.

Even a fabulous writer friend of mine whom we asked to edit this book couldn't muster the resolve to dive into this subject matter. He apologetically returned our check. That's how deeply we've all been conditioned to believe that this topic is off limits.

Unfortunately, even though hemorrhoids are such a common, annoying, and painful affliction, not much information is available about the subject, and what you do find is often confusing, scary, or outright inaccurate.

Ken and I intend this book to be the most complete source of helpful material on hemorrhoids and constipation available anywhere. Our approach is both medical and naturopathic. We provide the most up-to-date information about causes, solutions, and healing methods, and—perhaps more importantly—we talk about how to eliminate pain, discomfort, and suffering.

To complete this book, Ken researched hundreds of products, searched through volumes of reference materials, spoke with countless doctors and natural healing professionals, interviewed people suffering with these problems, and scoured the World Wide Web. Sherlock Holmes would have been proud. We've also tried to present the information in a form that's readable, easy to retain, and entertaining. As another friend once told me, nothing is so serious that you can't poke a little fun at it. After all, we're all in this together.

Coming up with a title for this book was one of the most difficult things I had to do. How would we call attention to these problems without offending anyone, and just how would we take such a sensitive issue and bring it out in the open. In the interest of pure entertainment, here are many of the names we came up with, some in the wee hours of the morning:

Hemorrhoids Be Gone; More Than You Ever Wanted to Know About Elimination; The Complete Guide to Your Guts (and Beyond); Don't Live With a Pain in the Butt; Simple Solutions to Painful Problems; Get Right, Get Regular; No Time for Constipation; Rid of 'Roids - Cured of Constipation, Hemorrhoids: A Gentle Cure; The Easy Elimination of Hemorrhoids and Constipation; When Hemorrhoids Attack, Fight Back; A Healthy End to Hemorrhoids and Constipation; An Owners Manual for Your Rear End; and, last but not least, The Handy Hemorrhoid Handbook!

We finally settled on our title *Put Hemorrhoids and Constipation Behind You,* since it seemed to convey exactly what this book is all about. So, as you start to read this book, know that there is valuable information in every chapter. Choose whatever method or suggestion feels comfortable to you, and get on the road to health and healing.

Chapter 1

There's Nothing to Be Ashamed Of!

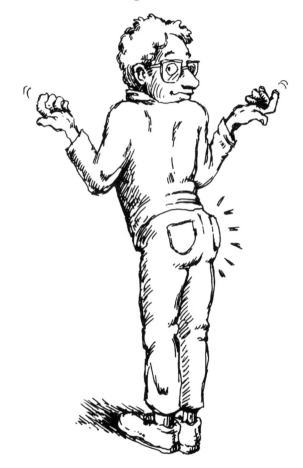

I want to begin with a simple message: "Don't be ashamed of your hemorrhoids or constipation!" If you feel embarrassed or frightened to speak about some of your 'nasty' symptoms, believe me, you're in good company. Over 80% of the United States' population has had colorectal symptoms, and most suffer in silence. Every year, 60,000 new cases of colorectal cancer are diagnosed, and this disease is itself related to 30,000 deaths per year! These statistics are staggering, and they tell us that something is very wrong!

We have inherited generations of distaste for mentioning certain subjects. Our tendency to remain silent has been respected and almost coveted, but unfortunately, has also stopped many of us from seeking the necessary help.

Not listening to our bodies' important messages and needs, has caused tremendous suffering and countless fatalities. As the baby-boomer generation, we have begun to develop an understanding of mind-body-spirit connections, and with this we can pave the way for new freedoms of expression and awareness.

In the last few years, I have been delighted to hear in soap operas, television sitcoms, and the movies, words like "bowels," "penis," "safe sex," and so on. The list has gradually grown, and this means we have the potential to give birth to a new era of taking responsibility for our personal health. To do so, we have to stop being ashamed of talking about our bodies and our problems.

Shame and embarrassment are common emotional responses to many types of menacing physical afflictions. Not unlike ostriches, we as humans tend to deny those problems that frighten us, particularly if these problems occur in the more intimate areas of our bodies, like our bowels. We minimize our discomfort and pain and don't discuss these sensitive issues with anyone, not even our doctors! This shame and embarrassment causes us to overlook indicators of debilitating and sometimes life threatening illnesses. We suffer grave, even fatal, consequences by burying our heads in the sand.

And shame is no easy foe! Take a moment to consider how powerful this feeling is. Has it ever led you to avoid certain actions even though you knew you would benefit from them? Or has it ever forced you to act hastily to make a decision for which you weren't ready? How many times have we fallen prey to peer pressure and did something we knew was wrong because we feared ridicule and embarrassment?

A keen example of our shame is cited in Sam's introduction: Preparation H™ is the second most frequently shoplifted item in pharmacies. What a potent illustration of how shame and embarrassment override our basic honesty! People would rather steal than admit they have hemorrhoids!

Sometimes I'm amazed by what things we choose to be ashamed of. We're embarrassed to discuss the natural process of eliminating our waste, yet we have no shame about stuffing our bodies with junk foods!

Stop hiding from the truth. Self-awareness is the key to prevention! Becoming aware of our physical problems puts us on the path to overcoming them. This is especially true in the context of our present day health care system, which puts more and more of the responsibility for our well being back on our own shoulders. The successful treatment of hemorrhoids and colon problems hinges on early detection. If shame or embarrassment leads us to neglect problems, they will go untreated. And we will have done ourselves irreparable harm. Even though it may be difficult, there's good reason to become aware of shameful feelings. Recognizing and stopping shame can actually help us explain symptoms to our doctors, thus avoiding more serious problems.

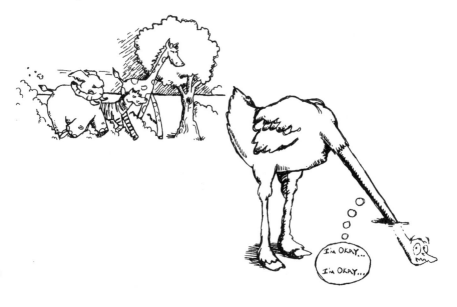

Unfortunately, doctors do not get courses in psychic diagnosis, nor is it their responsibility to call and ask about our health. It is even rare nowadays to find family physicians with firsthand and intimate knowledge of our family's health history. Consequently, we need to be aware of our own health and our own health history.

We need to know when to seek treatment and how to accurately describe our symptoms and concerns to our health care practitioners. It is imperative that we help our doctors by telling them all we know about ourselves. Otherwise, how can they respond with the appropriate care measures?

And what complicates the matter is the fact that there is an abundance of confusion about hemorrhoids and scant literature to reverse this situation. After dozens of hours spent surfing the World Wide Web, I found only two books on the topic! Let's put this in perspective: of over one million books listed, there were only *two* books on hemorrhoids! That's *ass*tounding (excuse the pun!), especially considering that there are well over 30,000 new publications printed each year on the topic of health.

The numbers just don't jive. Roughly 50% of our population has suffered from hemorrhoids, yet of the over 200 books that I used as research, few devoted more than a simple paragraph—or at most, one page—to the problem. Those that did cover the topic, typically said the same things!

Even more frightening was the fact that many authors writing about hemorrhoids said something to the effect - "Sometimes there is no reason for hemorrhoids." But this can't be; there is a reason for everything! Other authors argued that the most common cause of hemorrhoids was gravity. (To me, this sounds like an answer that's given when nothing else can be recognized!) These authors suggested that as we humans evolved from apes into beings that walked upright (thus placing more gravitational pressure on our behinds), we began to suffer more and more from hemorrhoids. In support of this theory, one author even writes, "After all, look at our family pets and animals; they don't suffer from hemorrhoids".

Well, maybe our family pets do suffer from hemorrhoids, but they just can't talk about it! Our pets usually don't get hemorrhoids because they're fed regulated foods with controlled portions of fiber and nutrients. They also drink when thirsty and get plenty of exercise!

As a youth, I remember witnessing a neighborhood dog dragging its butt across the lawn in an after-pooping ceremony. That sounds like a symptom of hemorrhoids to me! This dog was always fed from the table, eating the same food its owners ate. I was too young, though, and too embarrassed to ask if the whole family had bowel problems.

Perhaps I digress, but I do get angry when I hear supposedly knowledgeable people claim that there are "no reasons" for hemorrhoids. I'm convinced that the truth is these experts simply can't find the reasons. But I don't want any of you to settle for answers like "no reasons." I spend at least an hour and a half with my clients to find reasons, and later in this book, I'll teach you how to find reasons too!

Let me talk a little about how shame prevents us from understanding our bodies. I have been interviewing people about their health for almost 20 years, and it never ceases to amaze me that so many of us cannot describe our inner physical experience. For instance, a person once complained to me of stomach pain. "Where is the pain?" I asked. He responded, "Stomach!" and pointed below the belly button (which is not where our stomachs are). "What kind of pain are you experiencing?" I continued. But he could not describe the pain, even though I had prompted him. Was this person experiencing a sharp pain or a dull one? Was it an ache or was it radiating? He could not say, but if you and I want our healthcare practitioners to help us, we need to know how to describe our symptoms in detail. If we can do that, we've put ourselves on the path to recovery!

Another patient who complained to me of stomach discomfort could not bring himself to admit that his pain was from gas. It took me 45 minutes to find out that he had observed a change in his stool. Apparently, it had a flat side to it. To him, this change seemed "silly," so he buried the importance of this symptom. I surmised from our interview that his problem was due to internal hemorrhoids, and I then sent him to a doctor I highly esteem for a checkup. The diagnosis was Grade One hemorrhoids. (See Chapter 2 to find out exactly what Grade One hemorrhoids are.)

Within one week of treatment, this patient had no symptoms, and he thereby avoided a great deal of discomfort (not to mention lost time from work). If I had not pulled the needed information out of him, he may have been treated merely for gas, only to develop more severe hemorrhoids later down the road.

Doctors rely on us to tell them what is wrong, and most doctors don't have the time to spend 30 to 45 minutes teasing information out of us! We need to overcome our embarrassment and learn how to express our symptoms and discuss our problems. To me, this is simply saying that we need to grow up and become health-wise.

Colon problems can be painful! Pain, in fact, is one of our body's ways of talking to us. In a sense, it is our body's way of screaming, "HELP!" The message of pain tells us when something is wrong. Take, for example, when we pick up a scorching hot potato. The pain we feel is really the body yelling at us to drop that potato. Without it, we might hold onto the potato until it scorched our hands.

Or take another example. Say we start to feel discomfort in our tush. This discomfort is a message from our body that something may be wrong. Do we need to change our diet? Should we take in more fluids? Will a sitz bath help? Awareness of our body's messages is the key to prevention. If we "hear" what our body has to tell us, then we can take the needed steps to make ourselves healthier.

Review:

The first step in the treatment of hemorrhoids and other colon diseases begins with our minds. We must conquer our shame and allow ourselves to become aware of any physical changes that happen in our bodies, however slight, trivial, or silly they may seem. If we can do this, and then discuss our health problems with our health practitioners (no matter how delicate the subject may seem), we are on the road to recovery.

When describing our symptoms, we should be as detailed as possible. If we've done this, we can work with our healthcare practitioners to develop a course of action that will address our symptoms before they turn into something dangerous, perhaps even life-threatening.

Be assured, if you have a problem with hemorrhoids, constipation or if you have poor colon health, there is a reason, and reasons allow for solutions. You will want to find out the reason for your problems and work with your doctor and health professional to combat them. In the chapters to follow, I will help you recognize your specific problems, and explain how you can prevent them.

Chapter 2

What Are Hemorrhoids?[1]

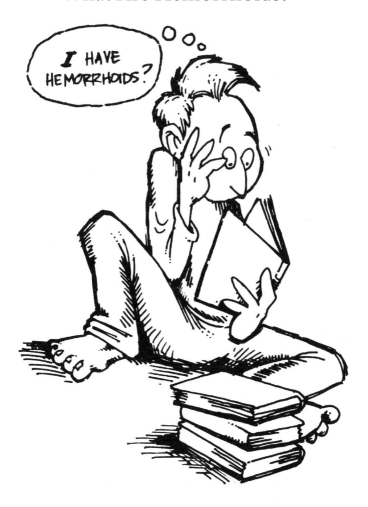

Believe it or not, everybody has hemorrhoids. "Oh No! Not me!" you say? Guess what? Hemorrhoids are simply veins around the anal opening.

[1] This chapter was written in collaboration with Steven Goldman, M.D., a surgeon and inventor of the "Comfy Cushion."

Your veins and your arteries are the passageways through which your heart distributes blood to every part of your body. Arteries deliver blood from your heart to the rest of your body, whereas veins return that blood from the rest of your body to your heart. The area around the rectum and anus happens to have large numbers of veins that all connect together, like a fish net. These veins are called the hemorrhoidal plexus.

Those veins that are inside the rectum are labeled the internal hemorrhoidal veins, and those around the outside of the opening are labeled the external hemorrhoidal veins. Normally these veins do not cause us a problem, but sometimes they become enlarged like the varicose veins people get in their legs.

The internal hemorrhoidal veins (those inside the rectum) can sometimes become so large that they protrude right out of the opening. When this happens these veins are called prolapsing hemorrhoids. (To prolapse means to fall or slip down.) Sometimes these hemorrhoids can become irritated and bleed.

Surprisingly, though, internal hemorrhoids may not hurt. They can bleed, they can cause a feeling of fullness, or they can even cause a discharge and itching; but they may not hurt. If pain is present, it is being caused by some other condition.

The external hemorrhoids (as opposed to the internal ones) usually cause no problem other than swelling. Occasionally, though, a blood clot can develop in an external hemorrhoid due to straining or prolonged sitting, and this indeed can be very painful. It is called a thrombosed hemorrhoid, and it feels like a hard, painful marble.

Depending on the degree of pain, thrombosed hemorrhoids can be treated with sitz baths, suppositories and topical ointments; and in most cases, they will go away within a week or so. If a thrombosed hemorrhoid is recurrent, or if it is painful enough to disrupt your daily activities (say, for example, you're unable to sit, walk or go to work), it will usually need to be removed in a doctor's office under local anesthesia.

The Classification of Hemorrhoids

Internal hemorrhoids are divided into four grades, according to their severity:

> _Grade One_ hemorrhoids are slightly enlarged and may bleed, but they do not prolapse.
>
> _Grade Two_ hemorrhoids prolapse with straining but recede on their own.
>
> _Grade Three_ hemorrhoids prolapse with straining, they bleed, and they have to be pushed back in place.
>
> _Grade Four_ hemorrhoids are so large that they protrude all the time and almost always bleed.

The Treatment of Hemorrhoids

There are many treatments for hemorrhoids, including stool softeners, injection therapy, banding, infrared coagulation, cryotherapy, surgery, and diet. The effectiveness of these treatments should be considered in light of the grade of hemorrhoids that are being treated. Let me explain each of these treatments and talk about what grade of hemorrhoids they are best suited for.

Stool softeners include suppositories and various ointments and creams. They are best suited for grade one hemorrhoids.

Injection therapy is similar to the treatment used to shrink varicose veins. It is usually used for grade one and grade two hemorrhoids. It entails the injection of a saline solution into the hemorrhoidal vein in order to shrink it. With this technique, the discomfort is usually minimal. The disadvantage is that the hemorrhoids usually return.

Banding is a technique used for hemorrhoids that have prolapsed, as is the case with grade three and grade four hemorrhoids. Banding entails placing a band (much like a rubber band) at the base or neck of a hemorrhoid to stop circulation.

This causes the hemorrhoid to shrivel up and fall off. Banding is a technique that has been used for many years. Because hemorrhoids usually return after banding, this treatment is usually considered a temporary measure, and it is used less and less. It also takes almost one week for the banding treatment to take effect, which can make it a very uncomfortable method

Infrared coagulation is a treatment which shows promising results for addressing grade one, grade two, and grade three hemorrhoids. It involves exposing the hemorrhoids to infrared light, which hopefully causes them to retreat back into the intestinal lining where they belong. It is a relatively non-invasive technique and only causes a minimum of discomfort (usually lasting a couple days).

Cryotherapy   is used for grade three and grade four hemorrhoids. In this treatment, the hemorrhoids are frozen so that they shrink and fall off. It causes some discomfort, which usually lasts for three to seven days. Because the hemorrhoids may return, this is often considered a temporary measure.

Various Treatments and the Grade of Hemorrhoids they Address

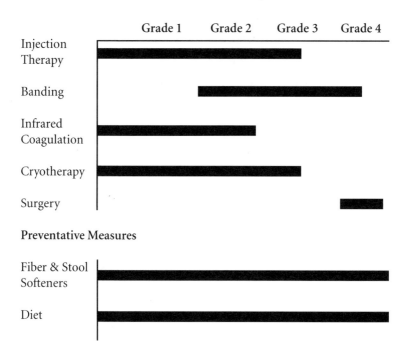

**Surgery (hemorrhoidectomy)** is usually considered a treatment of last resort. It is most appropriate for grade four hemorrhoids, which are often so large that they can only be treated by surgery.

This type of surgery would be performed in a hospital on an outpatient basis, and though it is not major surgery, it is nonetheless extremely uncomfortable. (Read Chapter 13 to learn just how uncomfortable surgery can be.) One will need pain pills for several days after the surgery. The discomfort makes it difficult to sit, and it is helpful to use a cushion to ease the pressure on the surgical area. See Appendix A for a discussion of this product.

**Diet** is the best preventative treatment for all grades of hemorrhoids. In Chapters 6 and 9, I discuss in detail how and what you should eat to avoid hemorrhoids and improve your overall health.

Chapter 3

A Quick Lesson on Fissures

You may wonder what your doctor means when he says you have fissures. Fissures are what you may have confused for hemorrhoids. They are slight tears that can occur in a hemorrhoid or in the intestinal wall itself. It is through this tear that blood droplets form and either appear in your stool or simply fall straight into the toilet bowl. Fissures, like hemorrhoids, are not dangerous in themselves, but they do indicate something is going wrong in your body and should be looked into as soon as possible.

The number one cause of fissures is hardened stool that scratches the surface of the intestinal lining and draws blood. As we will learn in Chapter 6, a diet low in fiber and fluids will cause stool to harden, and thus will commonly lead to fissures.

Another cause of fissures has to do with the digestive process. If our digestion is over or under active, then by the time food travels to the bottom of our colon, it may have become either too acidic or too alkaline. In either case, our rectum may get irritated and the lining at this juncture weakened. A simple scratch, perhaps by an undigested popcorn shell, may then open a fissure.

Fissures themselves are not a grave problem, yet they should be closely monitored by you and your physician. You should also have your doctor rule out the possibility that a more serious condition is causing blood to appear in your stool.

Such conditions include Irritable Bowel Syndrome (IBS), colitis, and Crohn's disease; and these can be quite serious!

The treatment of fissures is relatively simple, and there are various creams, ointments, and suppositories that provide effective relief and are available at most pharmacies.

These treatments, however, address only the symptoms (that is, your fissures), not the probable cause (your diet)! If you should chose one of these short-term treatments, be sure to ask your physician or pharmacist which is most appropriate for you. If you are curious about a long term approach, be sure to read about the Guidelines for Healthy Eating in Chapter 9.

Following this simple outline will encourage your body's natural healing process so that any tears you may have already developed, will soon mend. It will also help prevent fissures from reoccurring.

Chapter 4

Why Hemorrhoids
and Colon Problems Exist

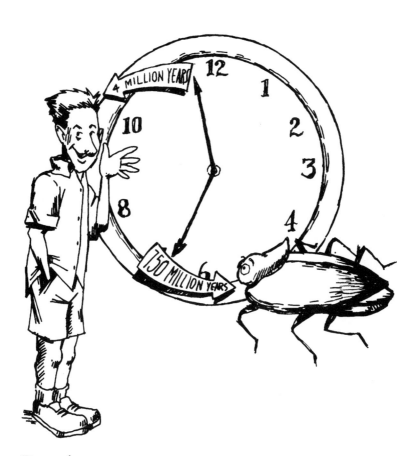

Premise

There are historical explanations for the tremendous rise of hemorrhoid and colon problems today. This chapter incorporates the work of both anthropologists and scientists, regarding the subject of Anthropological Nutrition. The premise is as follows: in the past four million years our human biology hasn't changed, but our life styles have. We humans were designed to feed and nourish ourselves in an environment that existed millions of years ago.

It's that simple!

Humans have had to adapt over time to a completely different way of existing; a totally different life style. In the millions of years gone by, we exercised our bodies daily in the pursuit of food. We *ran* for the hunt; we *walked* to *forage* for fruits and vegetables, and we *dug* deep in the ground for roots. We were also busy *digging* and *building* new cubbyholes in our caves and assembling our own furniture for shelter and comfort.

In contrast, today our pursuit of food consists of pushing a grocery cart down the isle of the closest supermarket. Our homes are built for us, and we pick out our furniture and have it delivered from local stores.

There is an expected side effect to all this convenience. We've actually encouraged most diseases that afflict us simply because we live and eat out of balance with nature. We've established unhealthy lifestyles relating to the way our bodies were originally designed.

Learning From History

We can now take a look at how and why we evolved as we did and learn to correct our bad habits. We can work our way back to optimum health!

Let's make this an exploration, and take a tour of human evolution to see where we took the misguided turn. The first hominids (beings who walk upright) appeared on earth somewhere between two and four million years ago. In fact, if we were to superimpose the entire evolution of our planet Earth onto a 12-hour clock face, as in the illustration, we would find that man has been on this planet the equivalent of two minutes. When you compare this to the cockroach, who showed up several hours before man (that is, around 750 million years ago), you can appreciate that humans are one of the most recent species to inhabit the Earth.

Paleoanthropologists believe, after the earliest hominids, Homo habilis (meaning "handyman") was the first hominid to develop tools for hunting and defending. Homo habilis appeared approximately two million years ago and was the first hunter-gatherer. Everything that the first hominids and Homo habilis ate was raw!

Moreover, these early hominids ate a predominately "vegan" diet. Bugs (and perhaps a few escargots) were the only non-plant life eaten. Today, our most basic biochemistry has *not* changed from our ancient ancestors and our bodies still remain best suited for a predominantly vegan diet.

This fact alone supports the premise that "we eat out of balance from our inherent design". Read on, and in Chapter 9, you'll find out that there is a way to eat meats and modern foods and still be true to our designs.

Does it matter that everything Homo habilis ate was raw? Yes! This is because all naturally occurring food contains enzymes.

Enzymes

What are enzymes? These are chemicals that aid us in digesting, absorbing, and utilizing all the nutrients in the foods we eat. But enzymes are sometimes destroyed in the processing and cooking of foods. Without enzymes, our body cannot make use of the nutrients in food, nor can we precisely digest our food. In addition, without proper and thorough digestion, our body cannot eliminate food waste efficiently. This increases the likelihood of constipation and hemorrhoids.

Unlike Homo habilis who ate raw, *enzyme rich foods*, we eat cooked or processed foods that are enzyme poor. This habit encourages constipation and hemorrhoids.

Does this mean we should eat all our food raw as Homo habilis did?

On one hand we know that cooking provides the benefit of destroying some pretty damaging organisms that live in our food. These organisms were responsible for shortening the lives of our ancestors.

On the other hand, we still have to assume that our original body design was to eat only raw enzyme rich foods. And since it would be both impracticable and distasteful for most of us to eat only raw food, the answer lies in the use of simple guidelines for healthy eating which are outlined in Chapter 9. By following these guidelines, you may enjoy all that modern life has to offer in a way that encourages healthy digestion and elimination.

Homo erectus

Homo erectus, living approximately 1½ million years ago, was the next step on the evolutionary ladder. Anthropologists and archeologists found that compared to "handyman," Homo erectus was taller, walked more upright, and had one-third more brain size. This bigger brain meant that Homo erectus could create and use more tools, and thus could eat a more varied diet. Accompanying these changes in brain size, human physiognomy also evolved. The shape of our teeth changed and we developed a more efficient jaw, so that we could now better incorporate meats into our diet. You might say that erectus was the predecessor of the "galloping gourmet".

However, the addition of more meat into the diet of early persons presented a digestive challenge. Since Homo erectus had no way to preserve or refrigerate meat, they were forced to gorge on large quantities of it when they were fortunate enough to make a kill. Yet, the human body finds it difficult to process a huge amount of food; our stomachs are only the size of a fist, and stomach starts to complain after two fists. A Homo erectus with indigestion would not have been a happy camper 1½ million years ago. The way erectus coped was by way of necessity; they had to eat lightly for as long as it took to bring home the bacon again. This allowed their stomach and entire digestive system to rest.

Homo erectus was furthermore able to cope with this digestive challenge because he led a physically strenuous life, which burned off the excess.

In addition, Homo erectus did not eat his meat at the same time he ate other foods. He gorged on meat alone when it was available and would eat fruits and vegetables at a different time. This also helped him to digest everything because of the enzymes contained in the natural foods.

Our stomachs produce digestive aids (enzymes). These enzymes, as it turns out, are food specific. Enzymes that break down meats are different than the enzymes that break down fruits or vegetables. Thus, in order for our bodies to digest food efficiently, it is best to eat only one type of food at a time. Homo erectus did this naturally; he kept proteins and carbohydrates out of his stomach simultaneously.

Neanderthals

About 130,000 years ago, Neanderthals arrived on the scene. Their brain size increased a third over that of Homo erectus. As a result of this increase, Neanderthals began using even more and more tools and utensils. They became more efficient hunters. Cooking became more prevalent. The Neanderthals began to use salt to preserve food, so they were able to make their lives a little easier. Because they were better hunters and could preserve foods, the Neanderthals ate more meat than Homo erectus. In addition, since the Neanderthal could preserve foods, Neanderthal, in general, ate more food than Homo erectus.

The Neanderthal probably was able to digest and assimilate their more varied and higher meat content diet for several reasons: They were very physically active, all their food was natural and unprocessed, they put foods in their stomachs separately (proper food combinations), and they did not eat dairy products which are impossible for the human body to completely digest.

Homo sapiens

Modern man—Homo sapiens, that is—finally popped up between 20,000 and 40,000 years ago. You and I are in this category and we are the smartest of earthly beings (although, sometimes I have to wonder). To avoid confusion, I'll draw a distinction between modern man (that is, Homo sapiens) and ultramodern persons (you and me). After all, modern man, when compared to you and me, really wasn't all that "modern."

As we evolved from modern man to ultramodern persons, our brainpower continued to increase. We increasingly cooked and processed foods; we ate a greater variety and greater quantities of food. We created more and more convenience devices, and our physical activity decreased.

Uh Oh! Sounds like trouble.

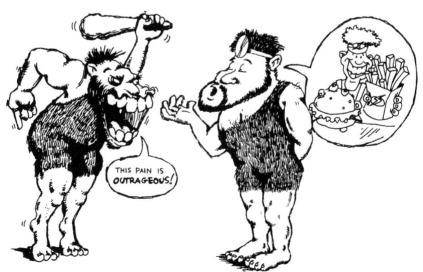

COULD BE ALL THE FAST FOODS- YOU'LL NEED MORE FIBER

The End Result.

One can clearly trace the evolving human eating habits from 'hunter/gatherer - eating only raw foods; to ultramodern mode of eating foods that have been precooked, overcooked, processed, polluted, preserved, distilled, broken down or— to sum it up in a word — modernized (for the worse).

We as ultramodern men and women are caught in a veritable quagmire of technological toxicity that would have discombobulated the digestive system of our ancestors.

In ancient times, we exercised all day just to find and catch the food needed to survive. Nowadays, most of us are competing in the "couch potato" Olympics. We have replaced hunting with a drive to the local supermarket, where we gather packets of foods that are barren of most vitamins and nutrients. Junky foods have become a way of life. We then cook this food, which further strips it of valuable enzymes and vitamins.

Making matters worse, we do not follow the cave dwellers rule of thumb, 'eat only when it is light out'! Today, we eat after the sun sets and sometimes late into the morning. But our stomachs weren't designed to handle large amounts of food before sleep, only to wake to a big breakfast.

Many of us eat large amounts of meat, and we eat meat, vegetables, grains and fruits together, instead of separately, as our ancient ancestors did. This had the effect of decreasing our body's ability to digest food and eliminate waste.

It should be no mystery then, as to why colon and rectal problems exist today. Our duty as individuals who want to live healthy and long lives, is to learn from our ancestors! Cave man knew (without even knowing it) what we've long since forgotten.

The Solution

But there is hope! Now that we know how we evolved and how our bodies were designed to work best, you and I are in a unique historical position to use our present knowledge to better our condition. Aren't our modern inventions, after all, meant to be life giving? Certainly not life-denying!

This book will utilize our past history and our present knowledge to provide you with solutions to improve your overall health, and ways to put your hemorrhoids and constipation behind you forever.

Chapter 5

The Stool Chapter

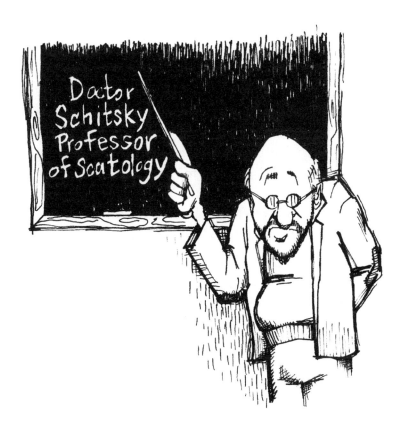

There are many signs that can tell us whether or not we're eating healthfully. One such sign, which most of us don't like to think about, is our stool (also known as scat, ca ca, poop, number two, plop, dump, log, and so on). It might amaze you, but there are whole sciences based on our stool.

This is because our waste can give us valuable information that will direct us to the optimum way to eat. In this chapter, you will learn to recognize your perfect stool. If you can get your own stool to be the color, buoyancy, size, texture, and shape of the perfect stools described below, you will be that much closer to having perfect eating habits, and this will help you maintain great colon health!

Note: I highly recommend you start keeping a food diary for this reason: if something unusual shows up in the toilet, you can look back to your diary and see if it correlates. I remember the first time I ate beets; the next day, after having my movement, I thought I was dying. The toilet bowl was filled with the red color of beets, and I thought this was my blood. A food diary will help keep you from making a similar mistake.

In your food diary, it may help you to keep track of these four items: what time you ate, what foods you ate, how large the portions were, and how you felt afterwards.

Color

Stool comes in many colors. It can be yellowish through gradations of green, brown and black. The color you want to aim for is a milk chocolate brown. If your stool is too dark or too light, this could mean one of two things. Either you're not digesting your food properly or the foods you ate the day before were light or dark in color. Your food diary should help you determine which is the case.

If your stool is ever black, this may be a bad sign and should be reported to your doctor. It often indicates the presence of blood in your stool. Stool that is yellow, green, or too dark might indicate improper liver function. The liver is responsible for producing bile, a digestive aid which is colored by pigments. Too little bile will give your stool a yellowish coloration; too much will cause it to turn dark green.

It's important to note that certain foods can also make your stool green, especially such foods as salads and green vegetables. If your stool happens to be dark green, check your food diary to see if you have eaten any spinach, kale (a type of lettuce), artichoke, asparagus, or other dark green vegetables lately. The color green may also indicate poor digestion of certain foods. You will want to check whether you're stool has undigested lettuce, spinach, or other green vegetables in it.

Undigested foods can make an appearance in stool for many reasons. Foods that are very high in fiber need to be chewed thoroughly for efficient digestion. Corn is the most salient example. If you don't chew corn completely (and that means each and every kernel), you will see the results in your toilet bowl.

Beets and sometimes celery may also make their presence known the next day in your bowl. Lettuce and other salad fixings, however, should be totally digested by the end of their journey, assuming your digestive system is working properly. Even peas eaten whole will get digested properly in a good digestive environment.

Those of you who like to eat the ends of asparagus may also see some hairy fibers at landings end. Some fruits that often turn up undigested in your stool—particularly if you eat them fast—include watermelon, mango, and certain berries. Most fruits, though, will digest completely if your digestive pipes are working correctly.

Buoyancy

Floaters and sinkers (no, this has nothing to do with baseball!) are two additional ways of describing our stool. A floating stool can be a good sign if your diet consists mostly of vegetables. The fibers in vegetables travel through the intestines and trap gas (which is lighter than water), thus floating our stool. Again, check your food diary to see if this is the case.

If you haven't eaten a great deal of vegetables lately, but your stool still floats, then you can surmise that there is undigested fat present. Fat, like gas, is lighter than water and will also float your stool.

Sometimes you will notice a fluffy, whitish border to your stool. This may be undigested fats, which show up in your stool as a foggy, milky residue. If you are a vegetarian or you happen to eat lots of vegetables, floating stool is an optimal scat. For meat eaters and people who take in lots of fats, floating stool may indicate a liver (or bile) problem. For those of us who eat both vegetables and meats, the optimal stool will sink to the bottom of the toilet.

Size

Size is another factor to consider when looking at our stool (though this is not a contest or a competition). For the most part, the size of our stool should be in direct proportion to how much we eat. But there are always exceptions to the rule.

Vegetarians, for instance, may have exceptionally large poops because of the amount of fiber they take in. When I was a vegan, I remember having stools over two feet long, sometimes twice a day (but I'm not bragging). Having been constipated most of my life, two-foot long stools were a dream come true.

For non-vegetarians, though, the rule holds, and stool size will vary in proportion to the intake of food. One should excrete nicely formed, six to ten inch logs. Two to three logs per sitting are considered normal and healthy, given a daily intake of around 2000 calories.

The width of your stool should equal the width of your colon, and this varies from person to person, of course (or should I say from colon to colon). To give you a rough guide, connect your middle finger to your thumb, and measure the resulting circumference. This should be the approximate width of your stool. (No need for toilet rulers or rubber gloves. Good old fashioned estimates will do just fine!)

Texture

The texture and formation of one's stool can be an important feature too. You've got your rough logs, smooth logs, hard packed logs, knarlies, rabbit turds, balls, bats, Mr. Softies, etc.. Again, not to be gross, but texture is a very important feature of a healthy bowel movement. Your stool's texture should correlate with what you eat. The food diary will be helpful.

The texture will also indicate your level of digestive efficiency. If you are eating lots of dense foods (like meats and fats) and a fair amount of vegetables, then stools that are Mr. Softies" are appropriate given your dietary situation. If you take vegetables out of your diet, however, and you still have Mr. Softies, then something is wrong.

In any case, Mr. Softies are not optimal because they indicate that your diet is too full of dense foods. The optimal texture of stool is somewhere between a rough log and smooth one (as if your stool were a clump of damp muddy earth). Any other texture indicates either a less than optimal diet or poor digestion.

Formation

The formation or shape of one's stool varies from person to person, digestive system to digestive system, and diet to diet. Because the last part of the colon has a squiggle to it (which is called the sigmoid) your morning bowel movement (which has usually had time to be molded by your colon) should usually have a slight S-curve at its very end.

The perfect stool for vegans should be a solid replica of the shape of the intestinal pipe. (To find out exactly what this shape is, refer to the diagram of the digestive system) To the compulsively oriented, the squiggle at the end of the bowel movement is considered the sign of a perfect stool!

Ease of Evacuation

The ease of our bowel movements is another delightful area of "crap criteria." It might be hard to believe, but the goal in terms of bowel movements is to sit down and move our waste within two minutes, if not sooner. (I call this the "two minute" rule.) The entire process of evacuation, from urge to evacuate to actual elimination, should take no longer than six minutes! If this does not sound like you (perhaps you're the type to bring a newspaper to the toilet), then you may have a way to go before having exemplary bowel movements. Chapters 6 and 9 will tell you what kind of foods you should eat to make the "two-minute" criterion a reality in your life.

Wiping

Another hard-to-believe statement about perfect bowel movements is that we should not have to wipe ourselves. Yes, you are reading correctly! This is the final goal of our bowel movement: to have no residue on the toilet paper. "How can this be?" you wonder. Well, think about this: God made humans approximately four million years ago, but humans have only had toilet paper since 1884 (when it was invented)! If your diet is perfect, you will have the ideal evacuation of your bowels with no mess.

Realize, though, that this a goal. Don't get discouraged if you're not there yet, but be sure to put yourself on the path to getting there. Everything will fall into place within a relatively short period of time if you begin eating right. Honest!

Chapter 6

Constipation: When Push Comes to Shove, Choose Natural Relief!

Constipation is not a root problem; it's a wake up call. It's an alarm that your body sounds when it needs to get your attention, and it does this by being a pain in the ass! Literally! But this "pain in the ass" is not the real problem, it's merely a symptom.

The real problem is something else that's going wrong with your body. It's just like when a smoke alarm goes off in your house: the problem isn't the sound of the alarm, the problem is the fire! The sounding of the smoke alarm is simply a sign or a symptom. But covering up a symptom (as we do when we take a laxative for our constipation) doesn't eliminate the problem.

In fact, it just worsens it, maybe even causing us to form hemorrhoids. What we need to do is treat the condition, not the symptom—put out the fire, not disable the alarm!.

If you have constipation, you need to proceed in a natural manner, eating the foods that your body was designed to eat. This will allow you to get out of your body's way, so to speak, so it can work on its own terms to heal itself. Constipation is easily remedied by eating a great diet; and a great diet includes lots of fiber, lots of fluids, and portions that are easy to digest.

THE DIGESTIVE SYSTEM

ALIMENTARY CANAL

Oral Cavity (a)
Pharynx (b)
Esophagus (c)
Stomach (d)
Small Intestine:
Duodenum (e)
Jejunum (f)
Ileum (g)
Largel Intestine:
Cecum (h)
Vermiform Appendix (h)
Ascending Colon (i)
Transverse Colon (j)
Descending Colon (k)
Sigmoid Colon (l)
Rectum (m)
Anal Canal (n)

ACCESSORY ORGANS

Teeth (o)
Tongue (p)
Salivary Glands:
Sublingual (q)
Submandibular (r)
Parotids (s)
Liver (t)
Gall Bladder (u)
Cystic Duct (u-1)
Common Bile (v)
Hepatic Duct (v-1)
Pancreas (w)
Spleen (x)
Descending Colon (k)
Sigmoid Colon (l)
Rectum (m)
Anal Canal (n)

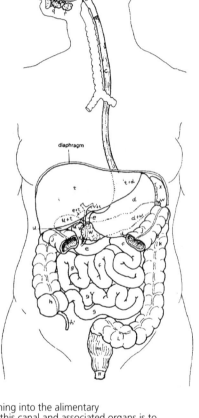

The digestive system consist of an *alimentary canal* with *accessory organs.* The canal starts with the oral cavity and continues to the anal canal. The major glands (liver, pancreas) have ducts opening into the alimentary canal. The principal function of this canal and associated organs is to prepare ingested food for absorption by the lining cells and the capillaries - both blood and lymphatic. In the mouth, the teeth and tongue pulverize the food with the aid of salivary gland secretions and the secretions of thousands of tiny mucous glands embedded in the lining (mucosa) of the oral and pharyngeal cavaties. The next site of chemical and mechanical digestion occurs in the stomach and continues through the small intestine. Only water, minerals, and certain vitamins are absorbed by the large intestine. Once absorbed, the nutrients are transported to the liver by the hepatic portal system where many of them are altered, stored, or metered out into the circulation via the hepatic veins. Nutrients are retrieved by the body's cells in the capillary circulation or by diffusion.

Kenneth Yasny, Ph.D. ©1997

I strongly advise that as long as you are not experiencing any medical emergencies you should attend to the root cause of your constipation rather than merely use medicines or vitamins to chase the symptoms away. I also suggest that if you do feel pain or fear, or if you do begin bleeding, contact your doctor immediately to get a better idea of what your problem is.

The Importance of Proper Digestion

To understand how to prevent the root causes of constipation, it helps to know a little about how the digestive system works. It is our alimentary canal (that is, our intestines) that digests and absorbs the nutrients in our foods and then eliminates the wastes. Food does not actually feed us, our alimentary canal, (circulation, metabolism, and cells) does! Without our intestines, we could never make use of nutrients from the many foods we so much enjoy.

When we experience constipation, this indicates that our digestive system is out of whack! There are many digestive issues that lead to constipation. Let me list a few:

- We may not have chewed our food well enough.

- We may have eaten too much food for our body to process efficiently.

- There may be too little or too much acid in our stomachs. This can be due to the fact that we've combined inappropriate food groups in our meals. (See Chapter 9 for an informative discussion of this.)

- Our liver or our pancreas may be overtaxed.

- The lining of our intestines may be irritated, thus causing a heavy layer of mucus to form.

- Our intestines may be in spasm.

- The movement of food through our alimentary canal may be too slow.

- We may not be eating enough vegetables in our diet, thus causing a poor colon environment (in which the levels of various intestinal bacteria become out of balance).

- Our intestinal muscles may be too weak.

In treating constipation, the goal is to get back to our natural states of being. We need to "lube" the tubes, speed up the flow, and bust through the logjam!

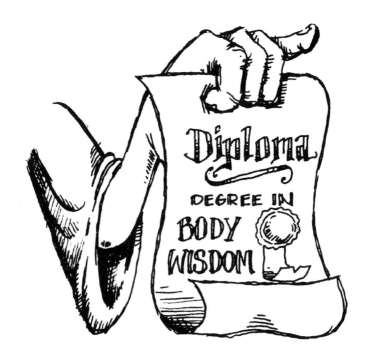

Body Wisdom

Usually all that is required to combat the old "sluggish bowel" syndrome is simple, uncomplicated "body wisdom." What is "body wisdom?" As I describe in my first book, *Talk To Me Body*, our bodies have a language all their own. If we listen to our bodies' symptoms, we will learn what it is we need to eat.

An incredible study I read almost 25 years ago, when I was in college, illustrates this point. Researchers took children from two to five years old and kept them in a school setting all day. They did not serve the children their meals, but instead spread out all types of healthy and unhealthy foods on tables. They then allowed the children to decide on their own what to eat. This study, which was conducted for a two-year period, found that the children chose a perfectly balanced menu all on their own. Now that is body wisdom!

Before I began my studies of nutritional science, this study touched me deeply and clued me into the concept that our bodies know more than our minds do. I promptly coined the term "body wisdom." I believe we all are born with this knowledge, though unfortunately most of us choose to ignore it.

Our symptoms, however, can lead us back to this knowledge. They can let us know what is good for us; and what is not. If we truly want to be free of constipation and hemorrhoids, we must regain our body wisdom.

The Symptoms of Constipation

The symptoms of constipation can be anywhere from annoying to incapacitating. We may suffer from bloating, distention, general discomfort, poor resistance to diseases, headaches, dry mouth, bad breath, physical weakness, dizziness, high or low appetite, cravings, mal absorption, allergies, blood sugar swings, mood swings, malnutrition, premenstrual syndrome, and low self esteem. This is a long list although it names only a few!

Several serious diseases can also stem from chronic constipation, including colitis (both bleeding and ulcerative), Crohn's disease, and diverticulitis. We should not take our constipation lightly! It can be a far reaching problem that is both horribly annoying and extremely serious.

Constipation can manifest in many different forms, and it's important that you identify exactly what type of constipation you are suffering from. The list below provides a description of several ways that constipation may manifest itself. Look it over and check the box to the left of those symptoms that affect you.

Remember, all the following are regarded as forms of constipation.

☐ Having an extreme urge to have a bowel movement, but being unable to move. This, of course, is our most common conception of what constitutes constipation.

☐ The inability to pass stool easily and at a natural pace. (The two minute rule from Chapter 5 applies here!)

☐ Irregularity. (I define irregularity as having less than one bowel movement per day, even if these movements are easy to pass).

☐ Hardened stools. (Even if we pass stool regularly, if our stools are hard, this constitutes constipation!)

☐ Malformed stools. (Stools that are flat on one side, for example, or stringy, or have knots in them.)

☐ A low volume of stool in respect to high volumes of food intake.

☐ Bowel movements that require some form of stimulant (such as coffee or some other type of laxative).

Note:	Keep in mind that the above examples are common symptoms, not disease states. There is no need to panic or worry if you have one of these symptoms; but do make sure that you do something about it.

Three Lessons for Treating Constipation

Now that we've identified what type of constipation you're suffering from, let's examine three simple lessons about how to treat constipation:

Lesson one: Moist food materials move through our systems better than hard or dry materials. (Pretty obvious, no?) It follows, then, that moist foods will often help us become regular. If we eat foods that absorb water (like high fiber foods), we will moisten the food inside our pipes and make our stool pass more easily.

Lesson two (taking lesson one a step further): The foods that best absorb water are those that are high in fiber content. Water-soaked fibers provide intestinal stimulation and lubrication that naturally propel food through our pipes in a proper and timely manner. Foods with the highest fiber content include non-starchy and mildly starchy vegetables, carbohydrates, and most unprocessed foods. (See the Food Classification Chart in Chapter 9 for a complete listing of foods that fall within these categories.)

Lesson three: Oils are slippery and lube all sorts of things (from car engines and door hinges to our intestines). To best "grease" our intestines and thus prevent constipation, we need to include a moderate amount of oils in our diet (mostly from the polyunsaturated and monounsaturated oil groups; see Chapter 9).

These three simple rules will help address any type of constipation. In the Chapter 9, we'll discuss how you can change the way you eat so that you are employing each of these rules to your benefit!

Chapter 7

Internal Spring Cleaning
Maintaining clean, rich blood and building a strong digestion

Dr. Charles Mayo, founder of the Mayo Clinic once said *"We are all afraid of germs because we are all ignorant of them. Germs are outside, what we should be afraid of is lowered resistance, which comes from within".*

You can't really control what germs come your way, unless you live in a biosphere. However, you are responsible for the "biosphere" inside your body. You decide what goes into it, when, and how much. You decide when (or if) you exercise, and how much you sleep. Some folks even say it's up to you to choose your own thoughts and emotions, which, needless to say, have an impact both obvious and subtle upon your amazing body.

Get Down to Basics
Nourishment comes from the foods we eat, and the only way to benefit from food nutrition is through efficient digestion. The nutrients are processed in the digestive system, and then need to be delivered throughout the body. This "special delivery" is accomplished by a remarkable distribution network known as the circulatory system, and is ongoing every second of your life.

The key player in circulation is, of course, our blood. The blood is like an army of couriers, or pizza delivery drivers – better yet, health food drivers, fearlessly racing throughout the canyons and hairpin turns of our arteries, veins and capillaries to bring the nourishment derived from food in the stomach to the rest of your hungry organs. These little nutrient "runners" work hard for you, so the least you can do is give them quality fuel.

Without a strong digestion which sets the stage for good absorption, the blood becomes weak. Digestion, absorption and circulation is nature's way of getting us the fuel and nutrients we need to run these bodies and stay healthy. Poor nutrition leads to "poor" or weak blood, and we begin to feel run-down. Unless we know better, this draggy feeling may lead us into poor lifestyle choices, such as increased stimulants (coffee, colas), increased sugar intake, and seeking out the dreaded "comfort" foods (you know, mashed potatoes with lots of butter, fettucini alfredo, ice cream, towers of drippy-warm cinnamon toast) when we in fact need just the opposite.

Digestion and Disease

The effects of weakened digestion are like a jagged rock in a river. After time, the rock will wear down. There is nothing in the river that maintains the rock to maintain its jagged edge, so it wears smooth. It's no secret that most Americans have strayed far from Nature's original eating plan for our species, and we stress and tax our resilient bodies with an array of habits which wear down and tear down our strength and resistance to disease. We strain or wear down our body's resources (like our natural enzymes) by overdoing everything. We eat too much, too often, and combine foods that really shouldn't go together (like meats and potatoes), and we eat foods not of the natural world (walk down the center aisles of any big supermarket and you'll see thousands of these, especially in the snack sections).

We overwork our systems until the body talks back to us (in symptoms). If you are lucky - the 'voice' is a cold or flu. If unlucky - this 'voice' is cancer. I ask you, What happens if you work too hard and push yourself beyond which is prudent? You get sick! Overworking the digestive systems will wear it out and get it sick. Weak digestion sets the stage for ill health.

Fasting

So, what do we do? Fast? Maybe. Maybe not! True, fasting has enjoyed a faddish popularity during the past thirty years or so. While fasting may be beneficial to the digestive system, it is not something to be taken lightly. A good fast is not just a matter of cranking up the Grateful Dead on the stereo and thinking pure thoughts, but must be entered into wisely and with preparation.

The dictionary defines fast as "rest". Rest is needed for repair. This is where Breakfast comes from…breaking the rest.

We've learned that our ancestors were forced to rest their digestion because food was not always consistently available. Most tribal peoples learned to cope with periodic famine— those woolly mammoth migrations could be hit or miss, you know. Luckily, things have progressed a bit since the Bronze Age, and our problem these days is just the reverse: too much food, always available.

Famine is never, to paraphrase Martha Stewart, a good thing, although controlled fasting may be helpful to adjusting your digestion. However, I have seen some people "rest" themselves right into sickness. You might say, "Too much of a good thing"? Remember that fasting forces the body to process and unload waste. Our bodies can literally choke on toxicity backing up trying to leave, not unlike Toxic Shock Syndrome. Our eliminative systems (skin, lungs, kidney, and bowels) cannot handle too much "detox" at one time. For this reason, a total fast (no nourishment) can be tricky, and not necessarily the best route for cleansing, I suggest a moderate, semi-fasting routine that will "cleanse" as well as support the entire alimentary canal and rehabilitate our digestive powers. This prevents nutritional breakdown, and makes the tummy and adjoining giblets feel calm, strong and happy.

Feeding and nourishing our entire body

Nowadays we have technology and knowledge on our side. With the help of vitamins, minerals, other supplements and vast information available on health, we can counteract the typically misguided modern lifestyle.

You now know that we get all of our nutrition from our digestive system, and that with a weakened system, we wear down. In the early 1900's Dr. Harvey Kellogg, founder of the Kellogg sanitarium of Battlecreek, Michigan and of the great cereal family stated, *"Of the 22,000 operations I have personally performed, I have never found a single normal colon."* This is especially staggering when you consider that the menu at the century's turn was almost exclusively "organic", less artificial, higher in natural fiber, with far less sugar and preservatives, than our present-day menu.

Even by calculating the lack of processing technology into diet of the roaring 20's, people abused their bodies to the point of ruining their digestive/absorptive systems by miscombining foods, eating too much, eating too late, eating more meats and fats than the body could handle and generally wearing the 'edges' down! Even then, Dr. Kellogg and later Dr. Mayo and many of his peers felt the urgency to care for the body's 'insides'.

The ONLY way to nourish our body is to keep our digestive pipes healthy.

Colon Cleansing Technology

Today we don't simply have fiber, we have colon cleansers, colon rinses, intestinal cleansers, vermifuge (anti-parasitics), etc. ad infinitum. My favorite cleansing supplements clean, support and nourish the body IN THE SAME WAY FOODS do!

Colon cleansers can either be gentle or rough. Don't panic— there's no black leather or body-piercing involved. In this context, gentle or rough refers to the actual fiber product you ingest. It may be made of soluble (gentle) fibers, or insoluble (rougher) fibers. Gentle fibers are particularly useful if one suffers from an Irritable Bowel Syndrome; rough fibers are great if you have sluggish bowel movements and need help with regularity.

Intestinal cleansers are groups of products that clean out and restore the general health and well-being of your alimentary canal. These products are designed to:

- Move out harmful waste
- Restore a healthy mucous lining
- Remove parasites and other nasty organisms
- Restore a healthy digestive environment
- Restore intestinal linings to health
- Restore normal levels of natural digestants
- Provide rest and recuperation for your intestinal track

The technology of intestinal cleansers will allow us to restore the natural balances. A sampling of these valuable tools are:

Vermifuge, herbs and supplements to detoxify and remove parasites. Garlic is perhaps the best-known vermifuge, with an ancient healing history. We're not sure about scaring off werewolves or curing the evil eye, but garlic, as well as onions, is a time-honored systemic cleanser.

Probiotic is a term that refers to intestinal floras that aid in our digestive environment, and is included in many of the finer intestinal cleansing products.

Fibers that simulate real food. These products feel familiar and natural to your body, and so create less disturbance.

Detoxing agents "trap" toxic waste (hopefully yours doesn't glow in the dark) so that your body can isolate these offending substances and quickly move them on down the line. Whew!

Of course, there is nothing that can take the place of good eating!

Enemas And Colonics

First, what are they? An enema is usually a 2 to 3 quart bag of water with a tube that's inserted into the rectum. It's designed to fill only the lower portion of your colon. A colonic machine is a device that gently runs 25 gallons of water in and out of your colon.

There are pluses and minuses to everything, enemas and colonics included. For instance, colonics can be a very useful tool in waste removal during fasting. Previously I stated, that fasting may force our bodies to work too hard.

As part of a fast, colonics and enemas ease this removal cycle. However, my personal opinion and professional observation lead me to the conclusion that colonics are not useful on a regular basis because they also remove vital minerals and upset flora balances— a case of throwing the baby out with the bath-water in digestive terms.

Enemas can be used in the same way as colonics. Enemas can also be used when we are sick. This an age-old remedy that my grandmother would suggest when I got sick as a child. Remember that we get sick when our eliminative systems are overloaded. Therefore, we can think of enemas as a method for ridding the body of wastes to allow our natural immune mechanisms to function more efficiently.

Colon Massage

Colon massage is a very simple method of helping your digestion and elimination. No, you don't need rubber gloves! Gentle, firm pressure on your abdomen stimulates circulation, relaxes your intestinal muscles, allows smoother, stronger digestive function, and can make you feel that all is right with the world.

A simple method of massage is to lay on your back with your knees in the air;

1. Begin with the tips of your fingers from both hands on the right hip side.
2. Using a circular motion press as deeply as you feel comfortable, and massage.
3. Continue this massaging motion in an upward position just below your ribs, then continue
4. across your abdomen just above your bellybutton then
5. downward to left hip.
6. You will make a short right turn, then down.

The more you practice colon massages, the more sensitive your fingers will become to your needs. You will also become adept at being able find your colon to massage or "de-kink" (yes, colons can get a little kinky) perceived blockages. This is a simple, completely natural and highly effective method of helping your elimination. Ahhh!

Feed Yourself

Finally, you are ready to read the next chapter! Find out how to put your hemorrhoids and constipation behind you forever, because if you do, you will enjoy great health and longevity. You will also be pleasantly surprised at how much better you will feel!

Chapter 8

All's Well that Ends Well
*Supplements, herbs, lotions
and all other kinds of wonderful stuff*

Too often, we only deal with symptoms of underlying problems in our lives. Those of you who work in corporate settings may have heard this phenomenon described as "reactive", versus "proactive". For good nutrition, comfortable digestion and more radiant overall health, it makes sense to support and protect your digestive system— also known as the alimentary canal— before you have symptoms, to prevent problems such as discomfort, impaired function, or other body-warning signs.

Constipation and Hemorrhoids don't come from nowhere. These uncomfortable conditions are the end result of problems within your entire digestive system. As the food you eat follows the path of the stomach, small intestine, colon, then finally the rectum, a problem in any of these parts of the body can ultimately cause constipation and hemorrhoids or something even worse. In this Chapter, we will talk not only about how to relieve constipation and hemorrhoids, but also how to better understand and maximize your own digestive system, in order to prevent future problems. Like the old song goes, the neck-bone's connected to the knee-bone! The chain of your digestion is only as strong as its weakest link, so you'll feel your best when all the components of your nutrition, digestion and elimination are considered as an inter-dependent system. Again to use a business metaphor— your body is a "team," so be sure that you're a team-player as well.

This information is organized so that you can easily track your symptoms and find relief. I make many references to specific products that you can find out more about in The Resource Directory at the end of this book. For convenience, you can even call *The Colon Health Society* to order all of your products from one source.

If you're in pain, discomfort or having a problem with hemorrhoids, constipation or other colon problems, this information will be a fast and easy guide for finding immediate relief. Product knowledge is every bit as important as exercising and eating "consciously" with health and nourishment in mind. After 20 years of working with people and their symptoms, I've come across many wonderful products that get the job done. You can easily obtain many of these specific products at your local health food store if they do not appear in the Resource Directory.

Identifying what's going on in your body is the first and most critical step. Until you have taken the time to relax and let yourself truly, fully feel your body's symptoms (as temporarily unpleasant as these may be), neither you nor your health care practitioner can effectively diagnose and treat the problem. Consider writing down a few notes about when and where the symptoms occurred. If you have a recurring digestive problem, consider keeping a journal or diary of symptoms, as a key to better understanding and prevention.

In order to obtain relief, follow these simple steps:

1. Grade your level of discomfort.
2. Pinpoint where in your body you are having the discomfort.
3. Identify the specific kind of discomfort you are experiencing.
4. Follow the suggestions below for your specific discomfort to find relief.

Grading Your Discomfort

Grade your discomfort as a level one, two or three. Level one discomfort is easy to ignore; level two discomfort is difficult to ignore, and level three discomfort is impossible to ignore. If you're presently only having mild discomfort (level one), you will be able to help all your problems by following the dietary suggestions in Chapter 9. If you're having level two or three discomfort, then continue below.

Pinpoint the Area of Discomfort

Many of us have lost the drumbeat of our own bodies. Our bodies talk to us all the time; we just have just forgotten how to listen. Much of the process of improving your health (not just digestive health, either) is remembering how to "hear" what your body says. Once you start paying attention, it's quite a chatterbox, by the way! Ask yourself "Exactly where is my pain or discomfort"? There are four basic areas of your alimentary canal (digestive system):

• stomach
• small intestine
• colon
• rectum

With help from the descriptions below, pinpoint in which of these areas you are experiencing your pain or discomfort.

Identify the Specific Kind of Discomfort

For example, a symptom such as bloating or distention — when your jeans cut at the waist, or you're a 42-year old man who feels pregnant— can simply be identified by locating the most accurate description of your discomfort. Most of the symptoms you are likely to experience can be found below in *The Solutions for Discomfort Sections* of this Chapter.

Suggestions

The suggestions will identify many general products. Immediately following the suggestions, are brands of products specific to helping you in the best way possible. These products are found in the Resource Directory at the end of the book.

Location, Location, Location

It's the key element in real estate, and it's key to appreciating the wonderful landscape of your body as well. Can you find your own organs?

Stomach - Place your fist, so the thumb knuckle is under your breastbone, and that's where your stomach is. It's actually a pouch of very strong muscles and its environment is acidic so it can break down food into a soft mush of nutrients. Sound yummy? The stomach prepares food for digestion in the small intestine.

Small intestines - Take your hand, and place your palm over your belly button and that's where these 32 feet of tubing are squiggled like wet spaghetti. They sit balled up inside the horseshoe shape of the colon. Here is where most of the digestion and absorption of nutrients happens. There are three parts to these pipes; they all prefer an alkaline environment.

Colon - The colon is approximately 6 feet long, is horseshoe-shaped, and absorbs excess fluids, minerals and some vitamins before elimination. It begins at your right hip at the ileocecal valve. After the ileocecal valve, it ascends, takes a left turn, and then descends. At the left hip it squiggles into the sigmoid, then onto the rectum. The environment is slightly acidic, and it has lots of friendly bacteria called flora.

Rectum - The rectum is at the end of the colon after the 'S' shaped sigmoid. If you don't know where to find it by now, you're in big trouble. It's a container for waste before elimination. The sphincter, which is a ring of muscles that closes off the rectum from the outside world, controls elimination. This sphincter is also known as the anus. Anal hygiene is very important. You may consider a bidet for this purpose (See the Resource Guide).

All good things—like last night's dinner—must come to an end!

THE DIGESTIVE SYSTEM

ALIMENTARY CANAL

Oral Cavity (a)
Pharynx (b)
Esophagus (c)
Stomach (d)
Small Intestine:
Duodenum (e)
Jejunum (f)
Ileum (g)
Largel Intestine:
Cecum (h)
Vermiform Appendix (h)
Ascending Colon (i)
Transverse Colon (j)
Descending Colon (k)
Sigmoid Colon (l)
Rectum (m)
Anal Canal (n)

ACCESSORY ORGANS

Teeth (o)
Tongue (p)
Salivary Glands:
Sublingual (q)
Submandibular (r)
Parotids (s)
Liver (t)
Gall Bladder (u)
Cystic Duct (u-1)
Common Bile (v)
Hepatic Duct (v-1)
Pancreas (w)
Spleen (x)
Descending Colon (k)
Sigmoid Colon (l)
Rectum (m)
Anal Canal (n)

The digestive system consist of an *alimentary canal* with *accessory organs.* The canal starts with the oral cavity and continues to the anal canal. The major glands (liver, pancreas) have ducts opening into the alimentary canal. The principal function of this canal and associated organs is to prepare ingested food for absorption by the lining cells and the capillaries - both blood and lymphatic. In the mouth, the teeth and tongue pulverize the food with the aid of salivary gland secretions and the secretions of thousands of tiny mucous glands embedded in the lining (mucosa) of the oral and pharyngeal cavaties. The next site of chemical and mechanical digestion occurs in the stomach and continues through the small intestine. Only water, minerals, and certain vitamins are absorbed by the large intestine. Once absorbed, the nutrients are transported to the liver by the hepatic portal system where many of them are altered, stored, or metered out into the circulation via the hepatic veins. Nutrients are retrieved by the body's cells in the capillary circulation or by diffusion.

diaphragm

Solutions for Discomfort or Pain in the Stomach

BURNING IN THE STOMACH can vary from a mild "simmering" feeling to searing pain. Your burning may be experienced at the top or bottom. Most folks would say that, after a major chips-and-salsa binge or a big bowl of green chili, that they have an "acid" stomach, when in fact the opposite is true. Burning sensations in the stomach are usually caused by too little stomach acid, so the food doesn't move out of your stomach into the small intestine quickly enough. Not only does the food sit in your stomach too long— so does the acid, causing irritation and burning.

Suggestions
- for immediate relief to neutralize the burning and protect or sooth the stomach lining from acid irritation, try aloe vera juice, calcium with magnesium tablets, or chlorophyll - either in powder, tablet or gel caplet form.
- for chronic burning, after the immediate burning has passed, eat more fiber, green veggies and brown rice.

Products
- Flex aloe vera juice, Ultimate Fiber, Bio Mucil, Kyogreen, Calcium from Molecular Biologics

BELCHING or burping, is caused by gas trapped in the stomach which creates pressure. The belching or burping is your body's attempt to relieve the pressure. Poor combinations of food, insufficient stomach acid, or overeating causes this problem.

Suggestions
- for immediate relief, first try the Betaine HCL tablets, then 3 sips of carbonated mineral water or any other

carbonated drink. If these solutions don't work, try drinking aloe vera juice.

- For chronic belching or burping, or belching or burping on an empty stomach, drink water, soup broth, eat toast or some protein, such as a hard-boiled egg.

Products

- Flex aloe vera juice, Molecular Biologics Calcium/Magnesium, Ultimate Oil

BLOATING/DISTENTION feels like there is a balloon in your stomach. It is the feeling that your belt is cinched way too tightly. Bloating or distention in the stomach is often caused by an irritated stomach lining or overeating.

Suggestions

- If you're bloated or distended on an empty stomach, this means your stomach lining is irritated. For immediate relief, try calcium tablets, papaya tablets, aloe vera juice, chlorophyll in powder, tablet, or gel caplet form, charcoal capsules or tablets, multi minerals or soup broth, all of which will sooth the irritation.
- If you're bloated or distended on a full stomach, don't eat for at least 2 hours. In addition, drinking aloe vera juice and using digestive enzymes will provide relief.

Products

- Molecular Biologics Calcium and Molecular Biologics Digestive Enzymes, Flex aloe vera juice, Trace Mineral Research, Secure, Kyogreen.

A DULL ACHE IN THE STOMACH is usually caused either by overeating, or eating something that cannot be digested, like milk or excess fat. The stomach muscles are forced to work too hard, and like any other muscle, they ache.

Suggestions

- If the dull ache is caused by overeating, for immediate relief, don't eat for at least two hours. In addition, aloe vera juice and digestive enzymes will help. If the dull ache is caused by eating something indigestible, then digestive enzymes will provide relief.
- For chronic stomachaches, use digestive aids, such as Betaine HCL, papaya tablets or digestive enzymes. In addition, try to eat only fruits and fiber drinks for one to three days.

Products

- Flex aloe vera juice, Molecular Biologics Digestive Enzymes, Ultimate Fiber, Super Cleanse, Perfect 7, Flora-Lyte, Bio Mucil, Living Foods

A SHARP PAIN IN THE STOMACH can stem from overeating or food allergies. But, if you have sharp pains in your stomach, particularly on an empty stomach, call your doctor, as this problem may indicate ulcers. A sharp pain on a full stomach is more likely to be caused by overeating or food allergies.

Suggestions

- for immediate relief, whether the cause is ulcers or overeating, aloe vera juice is important. If an ulcer is the probable cause, you should drink one cup of aloe and take calcium/magnesium tablets. If overeating is the cause, drink aloe vera juice, then eat lightly, sticking to fruits and green vegetables, and drink fiber drinks before your meal. Food allergies are commonly caused by dairy products, coffee, fried foods, eggplant, green pepper, tomato, potato or chocolate. To determine if your problem is caused by food allergies, try eliminating each of these foods from your diet, one by one, for four days, and see if that provides you with relief.

Product
- Flex aloe vera juice, Ultimate Cleanse, Bio Mucil, Living Foods, Trace Mineral Research

FOODS SITTING IN YOUR STOMACH which won't move. This problem is generally caused by overeating which over time weakens your stomach's ability to digest. To relieve this problem, we must repair the stomach and allow it to digest efficiently.

Suggestions
- For immediate relief, take aloe vera before meals, pancreatic digestive enzymes before meals, and use aloe vera and Betaine HCL tablets after meals.
- For chronic problems drink a fiber drink before breakfast with apple juice. In addition, make sure you eat small meals!

Product
- Molecular Biologics Digestive Enzymes, Ultimate Cleanse, Perfect 7, Bio Mucil, Living Food, Liquid Crystalloid Minerals

TIGHTNESS OR TENSION IN THE STOMACH can be caused by anxiety or stress, as well as overeating.

Suggestions
- Follow the same suggestions above. In addition, you may try meditation and relaxation exercises, get regular exercise, and use a Bodyslant to increase relaxation and circulation.

Product
- Flex aloe vera juice, Kyogreen, Molecular Biologics Digestive Enzymes, Ultimate Cleanse, Perfect 7, Bio Mucil, Living Food, Liquid Crystalloid Minerals, Bodyslant

RUMBLING (GROWLING) IN THE STOMACH can come from either too much or too little stomach acid. To relieve and prevent this problem, it is necessary to restore the proper acid level.

Suggestions
- if your stomach rumbles when empty, try fiber drinks, aloe vera juice, calcium/magnesium tablets or pancreatic enzymes.
- If your stomach rumbles when full, try Betaine HCL after food, aloe vera juice, soup broth, electrolyte drinks, or Liquid Crystalloid Minerals.

Products
- Flex aloe vera juice, Kyogreen, Molecular Biologics Digestive Enzymes and Molecular Biologics Calcium/Magnesium, Bodyslant for relaxation and circulation

Solutions for Discomfort or Pain in the Small Intestines.

PAIN OR RUMBLING IN THE SMALL INTESTINE, which may also be accompanied by flatulence, indicates gas or intestinal muscle spasms. These problems are often caused by an inability to digest, eating the wrong combinations of foods, eating too fast, or eating too much fiber.

Suggestions
- For immediate relief of these symptoms, try Betaine HCL after meals.
- For chronic problems try charcoal tablets between meals, Pancreatic digestive enzymes before meals, eat slowly, eat smaller meals, and eat more often. If necessary, use a fiber drink first thing in the morning.

Products
- Molecular Biologics Digestive Enzymes, Ultimate Cleanse, Super Cleanse, Bio Mucil

BURNING IN THE SMALL INTESTINES located to the right of your stomach, directly underneath your bottom most rib, is often a sign of a duodenal ulcer. Call your doctor immediately!

Suggestions
- For immediate relief (after calling your doctor) drink aloe vera juice and take calcium/magnesium tablets
- For chronic problems, eat small meals more often, take pancreatic enzymes before meals, try a fiber drink first thing in the morning.

Products
- Flex Aloe Vera Juice, Molecular Biologics calcium/magnesium and Molecular Biologics Digestive Enzymes, Kyogreen

A DULL ACHE IN THE SMALL INTESTINES indicates overused, weakened intestinal muscles, caused by a pattern of overeating, eating too late, or eating the wrong food combinations.

Suggestions
- To repair and strengthen your intestinal muscles, eat small meals, take pancreatic digestive enzymes before meals, aloe vera juice before meals, fiber and meal replacement drink for breakfast.

Products
- Molecular Biologics Digestive Enzymes, Flex aloe vera juice, pancreatic digestive enzymes, Ultimate Fiber, Living Food, Bio Mucil.

A SHARP PAIN IN THE SMALL INTESTINES below the stomach is caused by gas or muscle spasm.

Suggestions
- For immediate relief, try aloe vera juice, pancreatic digestive enzymes and minerals.
- In addition, for chronic problems, a fiber drink or meal replacement drink for breakfast. Avoiding irritants like coffee, alcohol, dairy, and processed sugar are helpful.

Products
- Flex aloe vera juice, Molecular Biologics Digestive Enzymes, Trace Minerals, Ultimate Fiber, Living Food, Molecular Biologics Bio Mucil

PAIN UNDER RIBS OR IN THE BELLY BUTTON is usually caused by gas accumulating in the small intestine. This problem generally stems from eating the wrong combinations of food, eating too much, eating too late, or food allergies.

Suggestions
- For immediate relief, try charcoal between meals, and pancreatic digestive enzymes before meals.
- For chronic problems, try pancreatic digestive enzymes, charcoal tablets or caplets between meals, and chlorophyll, either in powder, tablet or gel caplet form, probiotic powder, minerals, fiber drinks with meal replacement drink (Sometimes fiber drinks can create gas, however, this should only persist for a few days, then subside.)

Products
- Molecular Biologics Digestive Enzymes, Ultimate Fiber, Super Cleanse, Perfect 7, Living Food, Kyogreen, Probiotic, Bio Mucil, Flora-Lyte

PAIN IN THE HIP, LEFT OR RIGHT. If you experience pain in the right side of the hip, press firmly one inch over from your right hip; if there is extreme tenderness, call your doctor to rule out appendicitis. This pain can also indicate an irritation of the ileocecal valve, which your doctor can diagnose. Pain by the left hipbone usually indicates stress on the sigmoid at the end of your colon, which your doctor can diagnose.

Suggestions
- Once you have called your doctor to determine the problem, then take a fiber drink 3 times a day, preferably 20 minutes before meals, eat more fruit, vegetables and brown rice. If your bowel movement is regular, use pancreatic digestive enzymes. If your bowel movement is sluggish, use Betaine HCL after meals.

Product
- Molecular Biologics digestive enzymes and Molecular Biologics calcium, Flex Aloe Vera Juice, Kyogreen, Probiotic, Trace Mineral, Living Food, Ultimate Fiber, Molecular Biologics Bio Mucil

Solutions for Discomfort or Pain in the Colon

BLOATING, RUMBLING, AND/OR GAS IN THE COLON, which may be accompanied by flatulence, is usually caused by overeating, eating improper food combinations, eating too late, or nervousness.

Suggestions
- For immediate relief, try aloe vera juice, charcoal tablets or capsules between meals, digestive enzymes, fenugreek herbs or herb capsules, fennel herbs or herb capsules, probiotics.

- For chronic problems eat lightly for about three days avoiding raw food and use a small fiber drink three times a day. Also try Aloe vera juice, chlorophyll, either in powder, tablet or gel caplet form, probiotic powder, Calcium/magnesium tablet at night, and pancreatic enzymes if your bowel movement is regular or Betaine HCL if your bowel movement is sluggish.

Products
- Molecular Biologics digestive and Molecular Biologics calcium/magnesium tablets, Probiotic, Kyogreen, Flex aloe vera juice, Ultimate Fiber, Molecular Biologics Bio Mucil

PAIN THREE TO FOUR INCHES LEFT OF YOUR BELLY BUTTON is usually related to gas, constipation, sigmoid irritation or blockage.

Suggestions
- For immediate relief, try aloe vera juice, chlorophyll, either in powder, tablet or gel caplet form, and pancreatic enzymes if your bowel movement is regular, or Betaine HCL if your bowel movement is sluggish.
- For chronic problems, eat lightly for about three days avoiding raw food and use a small fiber drink three times a day. Also try aloe vera juice, chlorophyll, either in powder, tablet or gel caplet form, probiotic powder, and pancreatic enzymes if your bowel movement is regular or Betaine HCL if your bowel movement is sluggish.

Product
- Probiata, Flex Aloe Vera Juice, Kyogreen, Molecular Biologics Digestive Enzymes, Super Cleanse, Perfect 7, Bio Mucil, Living Food, Trace Minerals, Kyogreen, Probiotic.

PAIN TO THE RIGHT OF YOUR BELLY BUTTON. Call your doctor immediately to rule out appendix problems. If this problem is not appendix related, you may follow the same suggestions as for pain to the left of your belly button.

CRAMPS/CONTRACTIONS OR SPASMS/TWINGES in the colon can be related to constipation in mild cases, or colitis in more severe cases. Call your doctor to rule out colitis. Cramps may also be caused by improper electrolyte balance.

Suggestions
- For immediate relief, magnesium capsules or powder, aloe vera juice, chlorophyll, either in powder, tablet or gel caplet form , or massage the area .
- For chronic problems, follow the suggestions for immediate relief. In addition, try fiber drinks three times a day for three days, then once each morning or evening; trace minerals, meal replacement drinks, probiotics, and milk thistle. If you are constipated as well, try constipation homeopathics, gentle laxatives or laxative teas, Betane HCL after meals. If your stools are regular or loose, try rough fiber, pancreatic digestive enzymes before meals.

Products
- BHI Constipation Tablets, Molecular Biologics Digestive Enzymes, Magnesium Tablets, Trace Minerals, Agape Herbal Laxative Tea, Agape Herbal Laxative Tablets, Bio Mucil, Perfect 7, Ultimate Fiber, Ultimate Cleanse, Living Food, Seacure, Paeonia, BHI Hemorrhoid Suppositories, Flex Aloe Vera Juice, Trace Mineral Research, Liquid Crystalloid Minerals, Biodophilus, Milk Thistle, Probiata.

Solutions for Discomfort or Pain in the Rectum

BURNING IN THE RECTUM. This problem may be caused by nervousness/anxiety, food allergies, straining while eliminating, or possibly even parasites. It can also be caused by food traveling too fast through the digestive and elimination systems. Call your doctor and describe your symptoms.

Suggestions
• For immediate relief, drink aloe vera juice, take calcium/magnesium tablets, in addition, for chronic problems, eat small meals more often, take pancreatic enzymes before meals, and Kyolic with meals. Keep stool soft and regular.

Product
• BHI Constipation Tablets, BHI Paeonia, BHI Hemorrhoid suppositories, Flex aloe vera juice, Probiata, Kyolic, Ultimate Oil, Seacure, Pilex, Living Food, Clen-zone, Ultimate Cleanse, Molecular Biologics Stoneroot Complex and Molecular Biologics Hemorrhoidal Drops, Bodyslant, Comfy Cushion, Hemorrhoid Remedy, Hem-Tone, Vari-Care, Kyogreen, Trace Minerals, Lubidet.

BLEEDING IN THE RECTUM may be from a fissure or it could be from inside the colon as in the case of colitis.

Suggestions
• Call your doctor to rule out a more severe irritable bowel syndrome. For immediate relief, drink aloe vera and chlorophyll. Eat only cooked foods and lots of green vegetables, soup broth. Use suppositories, lotions, and tinctures. In addition, for chronic problems, use three fiber drinks per day and control your stress. Keep area clean.

Product
- BHI Constipation Tablets, BHI Paeonia, BHI Hemorrhoid Suppositories, Flex aloe vera juice, Probiata, Kyolic, Ultimate Oil, Seacure, Pilex, Living Food, Clenzone, Ultimate Cleanse, Molecular Biologics Stoneroot Complex and Hemorrhoidal Drops, Bodyslant, Comfy Cushion, Hemorrhoid Remedy, Hem-Tone, Vari-Care, Trace Minerals, Lubidet, Health Trek Hemorrhoid Jell.

ITCHING IN THE RECTUM is usually caused either by a food allergy, poor digestion, or parasites. Call your doctor to rule-out parasites. To relieve and prevent this problem,

Suggestions
- For immediate relief, you can use topical aloe vera and lotions. For chronic problems, avoid irritants like coffee, chocolate, dairy, processed sugar and drink aloe and chlorophyll. Keep area clean.

Products
- BHI Constipation Tablets, BHI Paeonia, BHI Hemorrhoid Suppositories, Flex aloe vera Juice, Probiata, Ultimate Oil, Seacure, Pilex, Living Food, Clen-zone, Ultimate Cleanse, Molecular Biologics Stoneroot Complex and Hemorrhoidal Drops, Trace Mineral Research, Kyogreen, Kyolic, Biodophilus Milk Thistle, Bodyslant, Comfy Cushion, Hemorrhoid Remedy, Hem-Tone, Vari-Care, Health Trek Hemorrhoid Jell.

SPASMS IN THE RECTUM are caused by too much waste, colitis, or a mineral imbalance. Spasms are usually the result of poor digestion and poor eating habits.

Suggestions
- To relieve and prevent this problem, eat lightly, eat small meals throughout the day, mineral tablets, drink lots of water and electrolyte beverages. Use fiber drinks, calcium/magnesium tablets before sleep.

Products - BHI Constipation Tablets, BHI Paeonia, BHI Hemorrhoid Suppositories, Flex aloe vera juice, Probiata, Ultimate Oil, Seacure, Pilex, Living Food, Clen-zone, Ultimate Cleanse, Bodyslant, Comfy Cushion, Hemorrhoid Remedy, Hem-Tone, Vari-Care, Kyolic, Trace Minerals, Health Trek Hemorrhoid Jell.

LEAKAGE OF WASTE FROM THE RECTUM . This problem usually occurs for the same reason as diarrhea. In addition, there is an irritation and weakening of the anal sphincter. Call your doctor to rule out a more severe irritable bowel syndrome.

Suggestions
- eat a simple diet of brown rice and vegetables and one piece of fruit per day. You may have up to 5 fiber drinks a day. Control your stress. Eat only cooked foods, lots of green vegetables, soup broth. Calcium citrate or lactate one tablet per hour if you have diarrhea. If diarrhea persists, call your doctor. Aloe vera can also be taken in an enema with chlorophyll and probiotics.

Products
- BHI Constipation Tablets, BHI Paeonia, BHI Hemorrhoid Suppositories, Flex aloe vera juice, Probiata, Ultimate Oil, Seacure, Pilex, Living Food, Clen-zone, Ultimate Cleanse, Molecular Biologics Stoneroot Complex and Hemorrhoidal Drops, Kyolic, Kyogreen, Trace Mineral Research, Ultimate Fiber, Bio Mucil, Liquid Crystalloid Minerals, Flora-Lyte, Cat's Claw, Bodyslant, Comfy Cushion, Hemorrhoid Remedy, Hem-Tone, Vari-Care.

INTERNAL HEMORRHOIDS are caused by poor eating habits and constipation.

Suggestions
*   Three or more fiber drinks a day if you are constipated. Increase fluid intake, mineral tablets, magnesium oxide/oratate/carbonate before sleep. Use topical salves and suppositories. The Zewa device may be of help.

Products
*   Pilex, BHI Constipation Tablets, BHI Paeonia, BHI Hemorrhoid Suppositories, Flex aloe vera juice, Probiata, Ultimate Oil, Seacure, Pilex, Living Food, Clen-Zone, Ultimate Cleanse, Molecular Biologics Stoneroot Complex, Molecular Biologics Hemorrhoidal Drops, Molecular Biologics digestive enzymes, Bodyslant, Herbal Comfort Products Remedy H, Trace Mineral Research, Perfect 7, Super Cleanse, Comfy Cushion, Hemorrhoid Remedy, Hem-Tone, Vari-Care, Health Trek Hemorrhoid Jell.

EXTERNAL HEMORRHOIDS are caused by poor eating habits and constipation.

Suggestions
*   Three or more fiber drinks a day if you are constipated. Increase fluid intake, mineral tablets, magnesium oxide/oratate/carbonate before sleep. Use topical salves and suppositories. The Zewa device may be of help. Speak to your doctor.

Products
*   Pilex, BHI Constipation Tablets, BHI Paeonia, BHI hemorrhoid suppositories, Flex Aloe Vera Juice, Probiata, Ultimate Oil, Seacure, Pilex, Living Food, Clen-zone, Ultimate Cleanse,

Molecular Biologics Stoneroot Complex and Hemorrhoidal Drops and digestive enzymes, Bodyslant, Herbal Comfort Products Remedy H, Trace Mineral Research, Perfect 7, Super Cleanse, Comfy Cushion, Hemorrhoid Remedy, Hem-Tone,Vari-Care, Health Trek Hemorrhoid Jell.

FISSURES are caused by constipation or diarrhea. They are slight tears in the rectum wall. Call your doctor to rule out a more severe irritable bowel syndrome.

Suggestions
- Control your stress. Aloe vera, chlorophyll. Eat cooked foods only lots of green vegetables, soup broth Three fiber drinks per day. Probiotics, try suppositories, lotions, and tinctures.

Products
- Pilex, BHI Constipation Tablets, BHI Paeonia, BHI Hemorrhoid Suppositories, Flex aloe vera juice, Probiata, Kyolic, Ultimate Oil, Seacure, Pilex, Living Food, Clenzone, Ultimate Cleanse, Molecular Biologics Stoneroot Complex and Hemorrhoidal Drops, Bodyslant, Comfy Cushion, Hemorrhoid Remedy, Hem-Tone, Vari-Care, Trace Minerals, Health Trek Hemorrhoid Jell.

Solutions for Other General Symptoms

DIARRHEA is caused by many factors which could originate in the small and large intestine.

Suggestions
- Control your stress. Aloe vera, chlorophyll. Eat only cooked foods and lots of green vegetables, soup broth. Calcium

citrate or lactate one tablet per hour until diarrhea stops. Three fiber drinks per day. If diarrhea persists call doctor.

Products

- Kyogreen, Probiata, Trace Minerals, Living Food, Seacure, Cat's claw, Bio Mucil, Biodophilus, Milk Thistle, Flora-Lyte, Liquid Crystal Minerals, Ultimate Fiber, Bodyslant

FATIGUE can come from weak digestion in any area. Over eating and food allergies may contribute.

Suggestions

- follow proper Food Guidelines and make sure you have an efficient digestive system. There are usually other symptoms accompanying fatigue. Follow the suggestions of those accompanying symptoms as they may be the real cause of your fatigue.

Products

- Kyogreen, Probiotic, Trace Minerals, Living Food, Seacure, Cat's claw, Bio Mucil, Biodophilus, Milk Thistle, Flora-Lyte, Liquid Crystal Minerals, Ultimate cleanse, Ultimate Fiber, Super Cleanse, Perfect 7, Flex aloe vera juice, Molecular Biologics Digestive Enzymes.

A CRAVING FOR SWEETS and hunger less than two hours after a meal indicates poor nutrient absorption.

Suggestions

- L-glutamine between meals, fiber drinks, probiotics, chlorophyll, aloe before meals, Betaine hcl, avoid milk products, coffee, alcohol, fried foods, and eat smaller size meals. Get regular exercise.

Products

- Ultimate Cleanse, Super Cleanse, Flex aloe vera juice, Perfect 7, Bio Mucil, Molecular Biologics Digestive Enzymes, Molecular Biologics Probiotic.

CONSTIPATION is a result of eating out of balance with nature usually relating to a weakened digestive system, poor food combining, and overeating.

Suggestions

- For relief of constipation, fiber drink before each meal, eat smaller portions more frequently, Betaine hcl after meals, magnesium oxide before sleep, probiotics. If necessary, use mild herbal laxatives, massage your colon.

Product

- Molecular Biologics Magnesium, Trace Minerals, Agape Herbal Laxative Tea or Herbal Laxative Tablets, Bio Mucil, Perfect 7, Ultimate Fiber, Ultimate Cleanse, Kyogreen, Living Food, Seacure, BHI Constipation Tablets

INCOMPLETE BOWEL MOVEMENTS are a feeling like you still have more waste to eliminate.

Suggestions

- Eat smaller portions more frequently if necessary. Betaine HCL after meals. Magnesium oxide before sleep. If necessary use mild herbal laxatives. Massage your colon, probiotics. Aloe vera, chlorophyll. Eat cooked foods, lots of green vegetables, soup broth and fluids. Three fiber drinks per day, aloe vera can also be taken as enema with chlorophyll, use three to five fiber drinks throughout the day, probiotics.

Products
- Molecular Biologics digestive enzymes, Molecular Biologics magnesium, Trace Minerals, Agape Herbal Laxative Tea or Herbal Laxative Tablets, Bio Mucil, Perfect 7, Ultimate Fiber, Ultimate Cleanse, Kyogreen, Living Food, Seacure, BHI Constipation Tablets

BLOOD IN STOOL – See fissure

MUCUS or fat on the stool usually relates to a mild to severe irritation of the lining. Maybe related to eating fats, dairy products or other food allergies. Mucus shows up as a milky fluff along the outside of the stool.

Suggestions
- Fiber drink with meal replacement each morning. Simple diet of cooked vegetables, brown rice and fruit. Probiotics. Call your doctor to rule out more severe problems.

Products
- BHI Constipation Tablets, Molecular Biologics Digestive Enzymes, Molecular Biologics Magnesium Tablets, Trace Minerals, Agape Herbal Laxative Tea, Agape Herbal Laxative Tablets, Bio Mucil, Perfect 7, Ultimate Fiber, Ultimate Cleanse, Living Food, Seacure, BHI Paeonia, BHI Hemorrhoid Suppositories, Flex aloe vera juice, Trace Mineral Research, Liquid Crystalloid Minerals, Biodophilus, Molecular Biologics Milk Thistle, Probiata.

Chapter 9

Guidelines for Healthy Eating

Diet

Let me begin this chapter by noting that the guidelines I describe below for eating healthfully are not a "diet" per se. Lately, the word *diet* has gotten a bad reputation. It would be helpful to avoid the term altogether, so we don't get too sidetracked by some of the misconceptions associated with this word. A goal of mine is to eventually get all people to define the word DIET as 'a healthful way to eat'.

My guidelines for healthy eating are not premised on fads, magic or any fly-by-night schemes. They are based on our current understanding of how to eat so that the human digestive system functions as efficiently as possible. These guidelines advise us to eat in the same natural manner that our ancestors did.

Once you begin observing these guidelines, you will notice many improvements in your general level of health, including an increased ease of weight control, improved immunity, increased stamina, and an increased resistance to allergies and colds. You may also be able to eliminate the worry of hemorrhoids and constipation from your life. You will be giving your body a long-needed opportunity to rest, heal and nourish itself.

First, know that following healthy guidelines will initiate the natural processes of self-cleansing and self-repairing; therefore, be aware that these processes often lead to side effects that *appear* to be negative by the unknowing person. I call these side effects "cleansing crises," and when they appear, they can be baffling.

Cleansing Crisis:

I remember the first time I experienced a cleansing crisis. I had just begun a diet of brown rice and vegetables (I felt great for about 3 months), and though I was eating what I considered a perfectly healthy diet, I got a tremendous asthma attack. I was livid!

When I began my own nutritional transformation, I was eating as healthy as I knew how, yet, there came a time when I felt terrible! The symptoms of this asthma attack, however, were short-lived, and afterwards, I felt better than I ever could remember. Since that time, I've not had another asthma attack, even though I'd had them regularly (2 times per week).

Cleansing crises, are good signs!

Don't be discouraged if they occur once you've begun following my guidelines for healthy eating. They can come in the form of asthma attacks, or—more typically—as mild cold or flu symptoms. Often they mimic symptoms that you've experienced in your past!

How to use Food Guidelines

Since everyone's body is different, YOU will need to adapt these guides to suit your particular needs. I encourage you to try them out and find what feels best.

Though my guidelines for healthy eating are founded on the eating habits of our ancient ancestors, this doesn't mean that we have to eat exactly as they did, hunting and foraging for food every day and eating only raw meats, vegetables, and fruits.

As ultramodern men and women, we've established that *our* hunting is done at the grocery store; and let's concede that the invention of fire is certainly a good thing - cooking foods can kill harmful parasites and bacteria. We don't have to abandon modern technology to be wholesome, but let's not forget our ancestral roots either!

What then, should we eat? Let us look at what most nutritional anthropologists believe the balanced diet was for cave persons. This will point us in the right direction.

Basic Guideline

From the research, it appears that approximately 70 percent of our calories should come from complex carbohydrates: foods like fruits, vegetables, grains and legumes (beans and peas), and 30 percent from meats and fats. *Estimates can be just as good as weights and measures when you get accustomed to the classification of foods.*

To be even more specific about how much meat and fat we should eat:
- 15% of our calories should consist of meats or some other protein source
- 11% should consist of oils, and
- 4% should consist of fats.

If you eat according to these proportions, your body will eventually work like a Swiss clock! Unfortunately, no one is going to figure out these percentages for you; you'll have to do this for yourself.

Enzymes

Enzymes are found in food, and are also manufactured by the body. They are simply chemicals that aid us in digesting, absorbing, and utilizing all the nutrients in the foods we eat.

Acid enzymes, it turns out, work in an acid environment (like the stomach). Alkaline enzymes, on the other hand, work in an alkaline environment (like the small intestine). Natural wisdom of early humans guided them to avoid the combination of meats (acidic foods) and carbohydrates (alkaline foods) in their meals.

Stool Analysis Theory

The Food Guidelines on the following pages coincide with what anthropologists analyzed from prehistoric mans' stool. This stool analysis revealed that cave people usually ate only *one food category* (such as proteins, carbohydrates or fats) at a meal.

This makes perfect sense considering how difficult it was to preserve food, and the difficulty on our digestive systems to break down more than one food group at a time. Biochemically speaking, carbohydrates (which are fruits, vegetables, breads and legumes for example), require alkaline enzymes to be digested; whereas proteins (all meats and eggs), require enzymes that do their job in an acid environment.

The simplest eating habit, then—that of dining on only one food group at a time—is the healthiest and most efficient. Isn't it a shame that such delicious foods as sandwiches and pizza, can be some of the worst foods for our digestive pipes?

If we, as ultramodern humans, heed the habits of our cave dweller ancestors, we should be in good shape.

Not only is it important that we balance our diet in terms of what foods we eat, but—as we've learned from the cave dwellers poop—combinations of foods matter as well. The cave dwellers ate simply! It isn't necessary that we obsessively adhere to this way of eating, but the closer we can get to it (and with the help of digestive enzymes) the better we will feel.

Seven Basic Guidelines

These guidelines will not only help to prevent constipation and hemorrhoids, but they will also promote the improvement of overall health and beauty.

Here's where it may be handy to review the **Food Classification Chart** and the **Sample Lunches and Dinners** at the end of this chapter. These will help you determine how to better balance your diet to eat the appropriate portions of complex carbohydrates, proteins, oils, and fats that are good for your body.

> *Guideline One:* Fruits should be eaten alone, either 20 minutes before any other meal or 1½ to 3 hours after. This is because simple carbohydrates (such as fruits and sugars) digest faster than any other food group. If you place easy to digest foods in your stomach on top of difficult to digest foods, be aware the simple foods will create gas. Simple foods want to leave your stomach fast. Complex foods, on the other hand, require more time to **fully** digest. Generally it takes a minimum of four to six hours for proteins and fats to leave the stomach; fruits and sugars take only 30 minutes to one hour. It's helpful to eat fruits before your meals. They prepare your stomach for the more complex foods to come. (Priming the pump, so to speak.)

Note: Your alimentary canal should process your food in approximately 12-16 hours. I call this "food transit time." It's the amount of the time it takes food to pass completely through your system.

Guideline Two: Proteins should be combined with only non-starchy or mildly starchy vegetables. Foods included in the protein category are fish, poultry, beef, and other meats. Eggs are also considered proteins. (Eggs are not dairy.) Because tofu digests like both proteins and carbohydrates, you can treat it as either proteins or carbohydrates when deciding what to combine with it.

Guideline Three: Carbohydrates (such as potatoes, beans, breads and rice), should be combined with only mildly starchy or non-starchy vegetables. Carbohydrates include these three basic groups from the **Food Classification Chart:** starchy vegetables, grains, and legumes.

Guideline Four: Fats and oils can be well combined with mildly starchy or non-starchy vegetables. I like to make a distinction between fats and oils. I consider fats to come from meat, dairy, and fried foods; and are solid at room temperature. These fats are usually the kind that can raise cholesterol levels. They are often referred to as saturated fats. (See the glossary for a more detailed explanation of saturated fats.) Oils, unlike fats, remain liquid at room temperature. An example of combining oils with mildly starchy vegetables is having a green vegetable salad with an oil based dressing. An example of combining fats with mildly starchy vegetables is having a green salad with a Ranch dressing.

Note: This is my own delineation between fats and oils. Technically speaking, oils are fats too. I make this distinction simply because it makes it easier for my patients to understand and separate what's best for them.

Guideline Five: It is best to avoid dairy foods because they are indigestible. (Milk, cheese, and any product made from milk is considered dairy.) It may come as a surprise to you, but only one being on the face of this earth can digest milk, and that being is a tiny organism that lives in the stomach of calves. Without that organism, calves themselves would be unable to digest their mothers' milk. In the human stomach, milk curdles and slows our digestion practically to a halt. To get an idea of what milk does to our digestive processes, compare the time it takes to exit milk from our stomach (from six to twelve hours) to the time it takes to digest fruits (30 minutes to an hour)! The difference is astounding. Fruits will take approximately 30 minutes to exit on an empty stomach. If you do eat dairy, it is well advised to combine it with lots or raw vegetables.

Guideline Six: Natural Desserts should be eaten alone, approximately 1½ to 3 hours after meals. When I say _natural_ deserts, I mean those dessert made with natural foods and sugars such as whole grains, honey, maple syrup, cane sugar, succanat, molasses, and so on. Even artificial sweeteners are acceptable when used in small amounts. Regular white table sugar, however, should be avoided as much as possible.

Guideline Seven: Your menu should limit the fats and saturated oils. (A good guide is to eat only one part saturated fat to every four parts unsaturated fat. For example, one tablespoon of butter to 4 tablespoons of olive oil.)

Monounsaturated and polyunsaturated oils should be used instead of saturated fats. As you've probably heard in recent media reports, olive oil is the best substitute for saturated fats. Many people have learned to enjoy olive oil instead of butter on such foods as baked potatoes, steamed vegetables, and bread.

HEALTHY FOOD COMBINATIONS

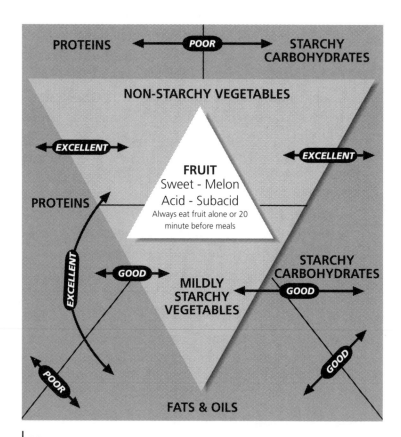

FOOD CLASSIFICATION CHART

Complex Carbohydrates

VEGETABLES - Potatoes (sweet, yams), Chestnuts, Squash (winter, acorn, hubbard, spaghetti, banana), Peas, Corn, Pumpkin, Jicama.
*Rice, Grains, and Beans also contain starches

GRAINS - Breads, Cereals, Buckwheat, Bulgur, Cornmeal, Flours, Wheat, Millet, Rices, Pastas.

LEGUMES - Beans (mung, lima, kidney, sprouted, garbanzo), Nuts, Seeds, Peas (split).

Proteins

FISH - All fish, plus Shrimp, Crab, and Lobster.

POULTRY - All birds

MEATS - Beef, Pork, Veal, Lamb, Cold Cuts.

EGGS

SOY - Tofu, Soy Cheese

Cheeses

HARD - Blue, Brie, American, Cheddar, Parmesan, Camembert, Swiss.

SOFT - Pot, Cottage, Sour, Yogurt, Riccotta, Rennetless, Raw Milk.

Desserts Made with naturally occurring sweeteners

- Muffins, Cakes (carrot, banana, etc.), Fruit Jell-O, Pies (fruit, yogurt), fruit and creme smoothies.
* Anything whole, non-stripped, little or no processing.

Fruits

SUBACID - Apples, Figs, Peaches, Plums, Nectarines, Cherries, Apricots, Papayas, Mangoes.

ACID - Oranges, Limes, Grapefruits, Pineapples, Pomegranates, Tart Berries, Grapes, Tomatoes.

SWEET - Bananas, Thompson Grapes, Persimmons, Dried Figs, Dates, Raisins, Prunes (most dried fruit).

MELONS - Crenshaw, Casaba, Cantaloupe, Water, HoneyDew, Christmas, Pie, Muskmelon.

Fats

SATURATED - Butter, Creme, Cream, Cheese, Egg Yolk, Lard, Milk, Ice Cream, Organ Meat, mostly animal.

UNSATURATED - Avocado, Corn, Sesame, Sunflower, Safflower, Olive, Margarine, Soybean, Peanut, mostly vegetable.

Mildly Starchy Vegetables

- Cauliflower, Beets, Carrots, Turnips, Rutabagas, Broccoli, Brussel Sprouts, Bell Peppers, Bamboo Shoots, Green Beans, Eggplant, Onion, Cucumber.

Non-Starchy Vegetables

- Lettuce, Parsley, Celery, Zucchini, Endive, Beet Greens, Spinach, Chives, Escarole, Garlic, Sprouted Seeds, Chicory, Cabbage, Radish, Collards, Chard, Bok Choy, Mustard Greens, Okra, Leeks, Watercress, Asparagus, Dandelion Greens, Tomatoes (acidic).

Kenneth Yasny, Ph.D. ©1997

ACID/ALKALINE FORMING FOODS

Fruits

ACID - Cranberries, Strawberries, Sour Fruits

ALKALINE - Apples, Bananas, Citrus Fruits, Grapes, Cherries, Peaches, Pears, Plums, Papaya, Pineapple, Berries, Apricots, Olives, Coconut, Dates

Vegetables

All vegetables are alkaline including potatoes, squash and parsnips

Grains

ACID - Brown Rice, Barley, Wheat, Oats, Rye

ALKALINE - Millet, Buckwheat, Corn, Sprouted Grains

Meat/Dairy

All vegetables are alkaline including potatoes, squash and parsnips

Nuts/Seeds

ACID - Cashews, Walnuts, Filberts, Peanuts, Pecans, Macadamia, Pumpkin, Sesame, Sunflower, Flax

ALKALINE - Almonds, Brazil nuts, All sprouted seeds

Beans/Peas

ACID - Lentils, Navy, Aduki, Kidney

ALKALINE - Soybeans, Limas, Sprouted beans

Sugars

All sugars are acid except honey

Oils

ACID - Nut oils, Butter, Cream

ALKALINE - Olive, Soy, Sesame, Sunflower, Corn, Safflower, Margarine

---

Important Notes:

If you are a **stressed** type person (A TYPE) who is high strung, eat mostly alkaline foods.

If you are a **relaxed** type person (B TYPE), and don't always feel under stress and pressure, use a balance of acid and alkaline foods.

Kenneth Yasny, Ph.D. ©1997

15 BREAKFAST SUGGESTIONS

1. **1/2 Papaya, 2 T. Granola**
2. **1/2 Grapefruit, 1/2 cup Granola/Grapenuts**
3. **1/2 cup Oats, 1/2 cup Granola** (cooked in water or water and apple juice)
4. **Stewed Fruit, (1 Tblsp. Yogurt)**
5. **Baked Apple, Cinnamon, (1 Tblsp. Yogurt)**
6. **Fruit Salad, 2 Poached Eggs, 1 pc. Whole Wheat Bread**
7. **2 or 3 Egg Omelette** (raw or cooked vegetables inside)
8. **1 cup Millet, Cinnamon, 25 Raisins** (cooked in water or water and apple juice)
9. **Bran Muffin, 1 Egg**
10. **1/2 Cantaloupe (1/3 Honey Dew Melon), 1 pc. Whole Wheat Bread**
11. **7 Grain Cereal, 25 Raisins** (cooked in water or water and apple juice)
12. **Cracked Wheat (Bulgur) 1 cup, 1/2 tsp. Tamari**
13. **Energy Drink -** 1/2 Papaya, l/4 cup Water, 1/4 cup Apple Juice, 1 tsp. Lemon, 1 Tblsp. Supplement Powder
14. **Eggs, Onions, Mushrooms**
15. **1/2 cup Granola, Fresh Fruit, Applesauce/or Apple Juice**

Solid Breakfast Suggestions

1. **Oats, Granola, Yogurt, Fruit (or any combination of these)**
2. **Fried Banana** (1 tsp. Oil, Water)**, Cinnamon, Almonds, Granola, Seeds, Chopped Ginger Root**
3. **French Toast -** Eggs, Non-Fat Milk, Vanilla, Cinnamon, use little Oil)
4.**Omelette, Vegetables, Bread (Sour Dough or Whole Wheat)**
5. **Eggs, Sliced Potatoes (baked)**
6. **Whole Wheat Pancakes, 1 Tblsp. Syrup, Fruit or Cinnamon**
7. **Whole Wheat Pancakes, Eggs**
8. **Eggs and Onions, Mushrooms, Whole Wheat Bread**

> *Important Notes:*
>
> Yogurt is a dairy food and should be avoided if digestive problems exist. Eaten occasionally, yogurt is fine.
>
> For breakfast, food combining can be eliminated if circumstances allow (i.e., Digestion is perfect and there is great hunger at breakfast in which a well-combined meal does not hold a person until lunch).

Kenneth Yasny, Ph.D. ©1997

17 LUNCH/DINNER SUGGESTIONS

1. **Brown Rice and Vegetables,** Spinach or Escarole Salad
2. **Winter Squash** (Acorn, Butternut)**, Peas and Carrots**
3. **Large Vegetables Salad and Tofu Dressing.**
4. **Vegetable Casserole -** Chopped Vegetables, Tomato Sauce, Seasonings (light sprinkling of Parmesan) and Salad
5. **Vegetable Soup (stew), Corn Bread** and Salad.
6. **Peppers stuffed with Rice** (Tomato Sauce optional) with Salad
7. **Grilled Tofu with Steamed Vegetables and/or Baked Eggplant** (baked with Soy Sauce and Lemon)
8. **Lentil, Bean or Slit Pea Soup** (with meat, if desired)
9. **Stuffed Baked Potato** (stuffed with Vegetables, in a little soy sauce and seasonings)
10. **Beans, Rice and Salad - (Tostada).**
11. **Zucchini stuffed with Rice** made with Galic, Onions and other Seasonings
12. **Sweet Potato, Soup (clear Chicken Broth with Vegetables Ok)** and Salad
13. **Fish, Vegetables** and Salad
14. **Chicken, Vegetables** and Salad
15. **Seafood, Vegetables** and Salad
16. **Large Vegetable Salad with one scoop of Tuna, Seafood or Egg Salad**
17. **Tofu Lasagna** (replace Pasta with Tofu - no cheese or Meat) and Salad.

NOTE:

1. Bread - Pasta - Potato or any starch is interchangeable.
2. Any protein is interchangeable.
3. Items listed for a meal may be omitted (salads for instance)

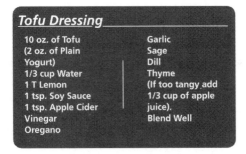

Tofu Dressing

10 oz. of Tofu (2 oz. of Plain Yogurt)	Garlic
	Sage
	Dill
1/3 cup Water	Thyme
1 T Lemon	(If too tangy add
1 tsp. Soy Sauce	1/3 cup of apple
1 tsp. Apple Cider Vinegar	juice).
Oregano	Blend Well

Kenneth Yasny, Ph.D. ©1997

Chapter 10

Hemorrhoidal Problems: Daily Living Issues

*(This chapter is rated U for uncomfortable!
Be warned that the language and visuals are graphic
and might make you uneasy. This is an opportunity
to practice getting over your shame.)*

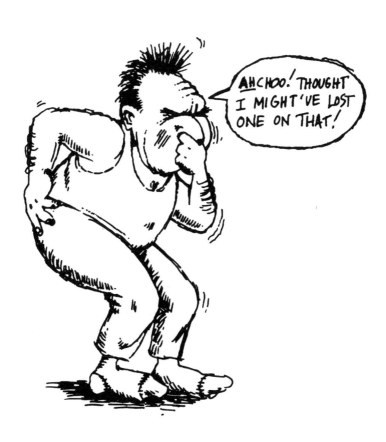

When we have hemorrhoids, the daily activities we take for granted become excruciatingly painful. Walking, sitting, bending, picking things up, sleeping, and even sneezing all become unpleasant.

There are additional problems associated with hemorrhoids, including gas, bloat, and difficulty urinating. How, then, can we live with hemorrhoids in a more comfortable fashion?

Let's begin with the most conspicuous difficulty we face when we have hemorrhoids:

How to have a bowel movement

For most of us with painful hemorrhoids, the thought of sitting on the toilet and eliminating waste is almost unbearable! We might even ask ourselves, "How can I possibly have a bowel movement with this condition?"

My first answer to this question is perhaps too obvious: don't acquire the condition to begin with! Prevention is always the best answer, and we've learned in the previous chapters just how we can eat to prevent this problem.

But let us say we have not been so fortunate as to prevent an outbreak of hemorrhoids. What do we do then? If an outbreak does occur, there are two secrets to easing discomfort and preventing injury.

These are: 1) have a soft movement, and
             2) relax!

We've already discussed the best way to have a soft movement: you should follow the dietary suggestions I lay out in Chapter 9.

The best way to relax is to breathe correctly and to become conscious of the muscle movements in your bowels. (These movements are called peristalsis.)

Breathing is one way that your body either holds on or lets go; and the goal in having your bowel movements, of course, is to let go! You also need to learn to control your abdominal muscles, so you can help the natural movement of your colon (that is, peristalsis). (See belly dancer).

When you get good at controlling these muscles, you will actually feel your bowel movement in progress. (See Chapter 11 on colon exercise to get a better idea of how your bowel muscles work and how you can get them in shape.)

Note: If you feel embarrassed or squeamish about this discussion, here are some helpful words of wisdom that my Grandmother gave to me: "It's your body, and there's nothing dirty about it!" Also, if you're embarrassed or afraid to touch the private areas like your rectum, remember that your body produces no substance that can't be fully cleansed by good old soap and water.

Speed of recovery is a very important factor when dealing with hemorrhoids, so you will want to overcome any embarrassment that may prevent you from doing what you need to do to heal your body.

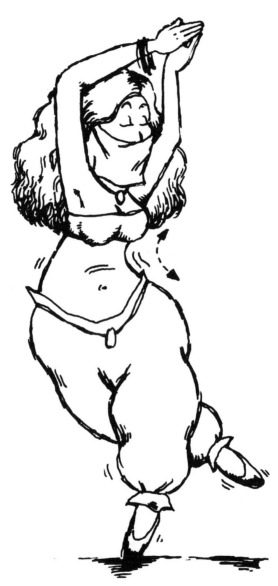

Here, then, is a general outline of how to achieve comfortable bowel movements even when you have hemorrhoids:

Phase one: **Have a soft movement!**

- Double your intake of fluids.

- Double your intake of high fiber foods (as outlined in Chapter 9), and decrease your intake of dense foods (meats and fats).

Phase two: Relax!

- Breathe correctly (that is, don't hold your breath)!

- Be conscious of your abdominal muscles. (See Chapter 11.)

What <u>Not</u> to Do…

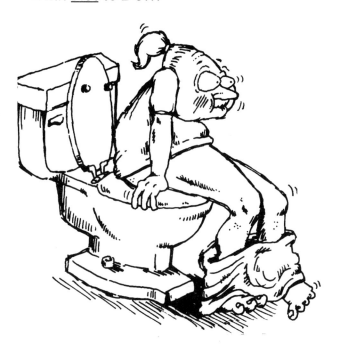

As I mentioned already, phase one—having a soft move-ment—is covered in detail in previous chapters (especially Chapter 6). Let's spend some time on phase two and dis-cuss the entire act of having a bowel movement so that it can be as comfortable and relaxed as possible. (I might add, too, that **practice makes perfect!**)

When we first attempt sitting to have a bowel movement, it is extremely helpful to have something to hold on to. This helps avoid strain. If you don't have anything to grasp, don't worry, the process is the same.

1). We begin the procedure standing,

2). with our legs together, and

3). our bodies facing away from the toilet.

Note: All bowel movements begin with tightening the butt muscle. This muscle, also known as the gluteus maxi-mus, is one of the body's largest muscles. (When I refer to tightening these butt muscles, I am also referring to the act of "sucking" in your anal sphincter. In this way, you keep hemorrhoids from popping out, which speeds healing.)

4). While you tighten your butt muscles, slowly sink toward the toilet seat, legs still to-gether, and—as the much as possible—hands touching the seat below to support your weight. Having your hands in this position will help ensure that you land on the toilet seat gently.

5). As you sit down on the toilet seat—still tightening your butt muscles and still supporting your weight with your hands—move your feet backwards toward the midpoint of the bowl. Slowly shift your body so that you angle away from the back of the toilet, with your weight balanced on the balls of your feet and your thighs. (Some weight can be balanced by your hands on the seat.) I call this the "motorcycle racer" position.

The Motorcycle Racer Position

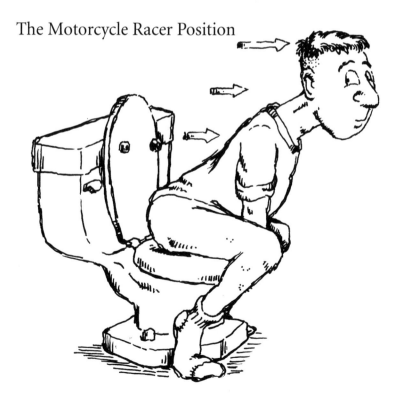

A variation of the motorcycle racer position is what I call the "gymnastic lift." This consists of achieving the same posture as in the motorcycle racer position, with the additional procedure of lifting most of your body weight off the toilet seat with your hands. The advantage of the gymnastic lift is that it further reduces pressure on your hemorrhoids. This is particularly desirable the more prolapsed your hemorrhoids are. Once you are in either the motorcycle racer or gymnastic lift position, you then relax and let go of your waste. It's that simple!

Note: If you are experiencing gas along with your hemorrhoids, you can comfortably release this gas by lying in a hot tub.

Helpful hints

Sometimes it may be necessary to aid the "letting go" process by lubricating the anus. A good way to do this is to use lubricants such as Vaseline, a commercially available hemorrhoidal ointment or an aloe or Vitamin 'E' based lotion. You can apply such lubricants with a Q-tip, some toilet tissue, or even your finger. Don't hesitate to apply a liberal amount. This is a good opportunity to push in any prolapsed hemorrhoids.

This will also help in case your stool is hard. Inserting the lubricant as high into the anal passage as possible will greatly ease your movements. Personally, I have found the use of lubricants to be a major help in dealing with bowel movements when my patients have had prolapsed hemorrhoids.

I have used lubricants not only to help push back a hemorrhoid, but also to release gas. Using the correct lubricants may also speed up healing. You may want to ask your health professional what is the best lubricant for your particular situation. (You can also check our Resource Directory in the back.)

Suppositories can also be of help for lubricating your bowel movements. The best way to use them is:

- to first lubricate the tip of the suppository,

- then bend over in as comfortable position as possible, and

- while holding the suppository in one hand, find your anal opening and insert the suppository.

Be sure to follow the path of the rectum gently and slowly. Here's a helpful trick: as you are inserting the suppository, feel for any protruding hemorrhoids and push them back in place. You may need to use more than one finger. Continue inserting the suppository until your sphincter reacts by "sucking" it up.

Note: You will want to become adept at this, because once you've experienced the feeling of the sucking sphincter, you'll be able to "suck" your hemorrhoids back into place, thereby accelerating the comfort and healing process. Though it may sound strange, it is actually a good idea to use a suppository when first practicing this action. This will allow you to experience that "sucking up" process. I can't stress enough the importance of getting this down pat. You will feel relief almost immediately!

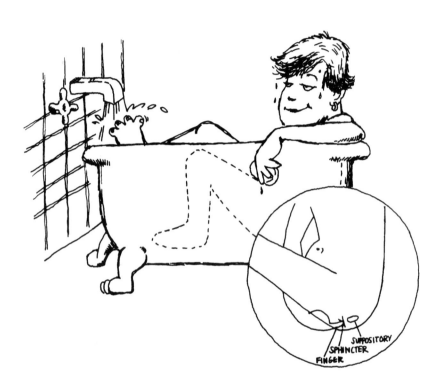

SUPPOSITORY
SPHINCTER
FINGER

The Pooping Position
When Business Is As Usual

Once you no longer have hemorrhoids, your goal for a perfect "pooping position" becomes entirely different. Instead of the motorcycle racer position or the gymnastic lift, you will want to adopt the same posture that our cave dwelling ancestors adopted; that of a simple squat. (See the Resource Directory under "The Welles Step" for a diagram of this position.)

The closest we can come to this position when sitting on the toilet is to proceed as follows: while sitting on the toilet, lean down, your arms across your knees, and point your toes so that your weight is on your tippy toes and elbows.

You will especially feel the benefit of this posture if you pull your knees towards your chest as you begin your movement. This will cause a slight rocking motion that will help push your stool out.

More Help

There are several mechanical aids that will help you get into this position. You can put telephone books under your toes, for example, to elevate the level of your knees; this is what gives you the squat position. There are also foot treadle devices that will help you accomplish this position. (Check the Resource Directory under "The Welles Step.")

Don't forget! It is important to keep your bottom area clean. I suggest that you use some over-the-counter preparations to keep your butt clean and to speed the healing of any swollen tissue.

The toilet tissue one uses is also very important. Never use hard or rough toilet tissue; only use soft brands. Soft toilet paper will help prevent re-injury. Soft, natural fiber is the best paper to use. Why take such good care of your bottom only to chaff it up with toilet paper.

Walking, bending, and sitting, must be done with great care when you have prolapsed hemorrhoids. The first step in accomplishing any activity is to prepare for that activity. Here are three easy steps to help you do that:

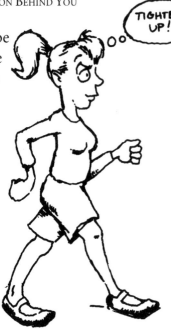

- Before you start an activity, begin squeezing your butt muscles as you suck up at the rectum.

- Next, as you initiate your activity, continue the squeezing of your butt muscles and the sucking up of your rectum.

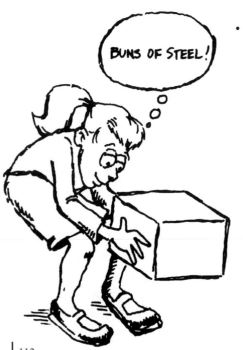

- Then, move as slowly and carefully as possible, so that you concentrate on keeping the correct posture while your perform the activity.

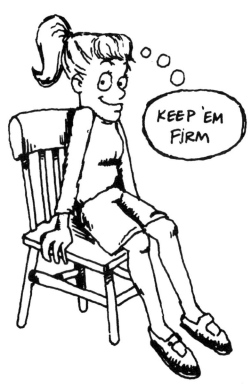

This three-step procedure becomes easier as you practice. Don't get discouraged if you can't seem to get the hang of this at first. Following this procedure for moving through your daily activities will make recovery faster more comfortable.

Chapter 11

Exercise for Colon Health

by James O'Connor[2]

*"If you don't find time for exercise now,
you will have to find time for illness later."*
-Wayne Pickering

Eating right is not the only thing you should do to improve your colon health; exercise is also very important. Our ancestors knew this. As we discussed in Chapter 4, our cave dwelling cousins exercised their bodies daily in the pursuit of food. They ran for the hunt; walked miles to forage for fruits and vegetables, and dug deep in the ground for roots. They also kept busy building additions to their abodes and assembling their own furniture for shelter and comfort.

Since the days of our cave dwelling cousins, we as ultra-modern humans have survived both the industrial and information revolutions, and as a result we live very sedentary lifestyles. We no longer exercise as regularly nor eat as healthily as our cave dwelling cousins did, and this has taken its toll or our bodies. (Remember, over 50% of the United States population gets constipation or hemorrhoids at some point in their lives!)

Once again, it's time for us to learn from our ancestors and get back to the basics. If we want good health (and that means good colon health too!), we need to exercise regu-

2 James O'Connor is an exercise physiologist specializing in colon health and a graduate of the University of Wisconsin. He has been in private practice for 12 years.

larly. Usually when we hear about exercise, we think of boring, strenuous, and painful workouts. But that simply need not be the case. A ten-year study concluded in 1996 by the Surgeon General and the Center for Disease Control in Atlanta revealed that an exercise regimen didn't need to be strenuous to be health giving. It simply needed to provide a moderate workout of the cardiovascular system at least three times a week.

This same ten-year study revealed that colon health is one of the major beneficiaries of a regular exercise regimen. Our alimentary tract is comprised of smooth muscle tissue that moves food through our body by continuously contracting and relaxing. (This process is technically known as peristalsis.) The muscle tissue in our alimentary tract, like the muscle tissue throughout the rest our body, works best when it is in top physical condition, and the way to get this muscle tissue into top physical condition is to exercise regularly.

When we exercise, our heart muscle saturates the billions of cells in our body with blood and lymph. This benefits all our body's organs, not just our muscles. The specific way our alimentary canal benefits is that it begins to digest and absorb food more efficiently and more speedily.

This not only helps prevent such maladies as hemorrhoids and constipation, but it also decreases the likelihood of colon cancer. I think you'll be amazed at the beneficial effects of a regular exercise program. (As an experiment, try exercising one hour before a meal and just watch how this improves your digestive functioning!)

A Seven-Step Exercise Program for Optimal Colon Health

Now let's discuss a simple seven-step exercise program that will help you maintain excellent general health and excellent colon health. If you follow each of these steps, you'll set yourself up for an exercise experience that will yield noticeable results in little time.

Step One: Contact your physician.

Before you begin any exercise program, you should always contact your physician. Generally, a physical is all you will need. You will also want to find out

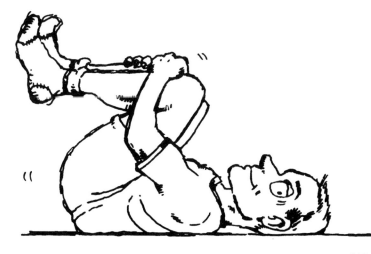

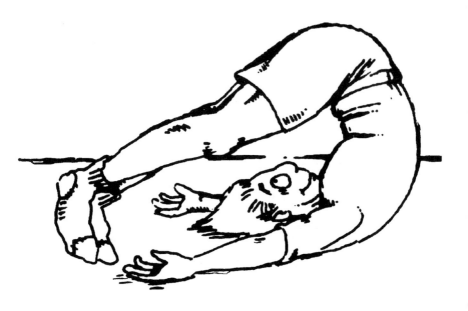

from your doctor if you have any medical limitations that you should keep in mind when designing a personal exercise program.

Step Two: Consult a qualified exercise physiologist.

The word "qualified" here is extremely important! A qualified exercise physiologist will have a degree specifically in exercise physiology. They should also have experience. Be sure to check out your exercise physiologist's background.

A good way to do this is to ask them for their résumé. Another way to go is to ask friends for referrals. There are agencies that will provide referrals. Also, colleges that offer programs in exercise physiology (such as UCLA) can provide information.

Once you have found a good exercise physiologist, here's what they should do for you: take your medical history, evaluate your current physical condition, and help you determine your exercise goals. They should also work closely with your doctor to help you accomplish these goals.

Please, don't adopt the exercise theories you hear from friends or read in magazines! Rely on a professional. This is crucial; everyone's exercise program is different, due to the fact that each of us has specific medical issues and our own individual goals. By working with a professional, you'll receive the best guidance available while saving yourself valuable time.

Step Three: Write down your specific health and exercise goals.

Writing down your goals is a powerful way of committing yourself to your physical program. Everyday, you should take out your goals, look at them, and recite them to yourself. Set realistic, short term goals. (Remember, physical activity need not be strenuous to get results.) As soon as you start your program, you will be helping your colon health. And again, don't listen to your friends or to magazines; listen to professionals. Only they know what's best for you.

Step Four: Make sure your program includes a cardio-vascular component.

You will need to exercise your cardiovascular system a minimum of three days per week, with each session lasting at least 20 minutes. Your goal during these exercise sessions is to get your heart pumping at approximately 60 to 75 percent its full capacity.

This is what I call the "target zone," and it can be determined by taking your age, subtracting it from 220, and then multiplying this number by .60 (for the low end of your zone) and .75 (for the high end). This will give you a heart-rate range to shoot for. (You can measure your current heart rate or your heart rate during exercise by simply feeling for your pulse on your wrist or neck, counting how many times your heart beats in ten seconds, and multiplying by six).

Walking and swimming are probably the two best cardiovascular exercise, but don't limit yourself to these. Choose activities you enjoy!

Step Five: Make sure your program includes a strength training component.

Strength training is the best exercise modality for losing body fat and for strengthening muscles and bones. Research states that for the best results in muscle strengthening, you only need to exercise one set of muscle groups to the point of exhaustion on two nonconsecutive days per week. Research has also shown that strength training increases gastrointestinal transit time (that is, the time it takes food to go from you mouth to your bowels), and thus improves colon health.

When you do strength exercises, each repetition should consist of a slow and controlled, full-range motion. Two seconds should be dedicated for the positive motion, and four seconds for the negative motion.

Positive motion means you are exerting force to move the weight away from its original position, whereas negative motion means that you are allowing gravity to move the weight back to its original position. Strength training should be done by everyone, no matter what age (unless, of course, one has a medical limitation).

Step Six: Make sure your program includes flexibility training.

There are two very important reasons for doing flexibility training. First, it is a wonderful way to relax, and the process of relaxation will help you develop an awareness of the link between mind and body. The better you understand this link, the better you will become at preventing constipation and hemorrhoids.

Second, flexibility exercises are a great way to warm up the body before doing other physical activities, such as cardiovascular exercises or strength training. Flexibility training, by making the joints more resilient and by transporting blood to different parts of the body, greatly reduces the likelihood of injury. Flexibility stretches can also have a soothing effect on the intestines, which helps peristalsis.

Yoga, pilates, and stretching are all excellent ways to achieve flexibility training. When you do stretches, these should be static (with no bouncing), and each stretch should be held for a minimum for 30 seconds. You should stretch before and after every exercise session (whether these exercises are cardiovascular or for strength training). A few good flexibility stretches for colon health are illustrated in this chapter. (For more extensive descriptions please refer to the workbook.)

There are also certain equipment aids which can assist you in accomplishing your flexibility goals. Please refer to the workbook for more information on these aids.

Step Seven: Stay consistent!

If you miss a day, get back on the program as soon as possible. If it helps, remind yourself every day that exercise is of tremendous benefit for healing your colon problems.

Clearly, exercise is beneficial not only for your colon health, but for your entire lifestyle! You will feel benefits from an exercise program very quickly, and you needn't engage in strenuous exercises to receive those benefits. Did you know that every week you have 168 hours at your disposal, and you only need to spend 1 to 1.5 of these hours doing exercise (that's less than 1% of your time)? Isn't your health worth it?

Just remember to consult a doctor and a professional exercise physiologist about your exercise program before you begin. This will ensure that you receive the best results in the least time.

Chapter 12

Questions and Answers

Throughout my career as a nutritionist, my clients have come to me with many questions and concerns about hemorrhoids and constipation. In this chapter, I review many of their most common and pressing questions. You will probably find many questions here that you yourself have wanted to ask. I hope you find comfort and guidance in the answers below.

If you have further questions after reading this chapter, please contact your local health practitioner. You can also contact *The Colon Health Society* mentioned at the end of this book.

Are hemorrhoids cancerous or life threatening?

No. Hemorrhoids are usually no more than discomforting and inconvenient. If hemorrhoids get severe, however, they can become quite painful and should be attended to immediately.

Will I need surgery?

If you attend to your colon problems in their early stages, it is very unlikely that you will need surgery. If your discomfort becomes is too great, however, you should seek the aid of a specialist to gauge the seriousness of the problem. Still, you may not need surgery. This really depends on the severity of your problem.

Should your physician determine that you do need surgery, there's no reason for concern. The surgery is simple and is usually performed on an outpatient basis. You should prepare yourself, however, for extreme discomfort after this treatment. (Read Chapter 13 to learn just how uncomfortable surgery can be.) You will probably need pain pills for several days following surgery, and it will be difficult to sit. (See Appendix C for a discussion of the "Comfy Cushion," a device that makes sitting after this surgery much less painful.)

Before you do have surgery, you should learn as much about your symptoms and problems as possible; then you'll be able to make an educated decision about the course of treatment. You will want to explore all the alternatives thoroughly.

Will I get hemorrhoids as a result of pregnancy?

Most women (80%) get hemorrhoids as a result of pregnancy. This does not mean, though, that you'll definitely get hemorrhoids. If you take the necessary preventive measures, you will greatly reduce this likelihood.

The key to avoiding hemorrhoids when you're pregnant is to regulate your bowels. If your stools are too firm or too hard, you need to increase your fiber and fluid intake (as we discussed in Chapters 6 and 9). To get through pregnancy with hemorrhoids, you may want to use various creams and ointments (available at your local drugstore) to help you keep your tissue healthy. Hemorrhoids can also be caused by a weak veins system. A good healthy diet, one high in bioflavonoids, will often counteract this problem .

Why is it hard to find information on hemorrhoids?

Until recently, hemorrhoids and our bowels generally have been topics of non-discussion even in the literature on nutrition and health. This has changed, however, due to a tremendous rise in bowel problems in the past half century. Finally, society is beginning to recognize and deal with health issues pertaining to our bowels. And because we are currently seeing 60 thousand new cases of colon cancer every year, we will continue to hear more and more about these issues.

Currently, the books available on hemorrhoids and colon health, say very little, and most of what is said is not up to date. When I did my research, I found very little new material. Hopefully, as people become more concerned about these issues, greater research will be conducted, and we will learn more about how to prevent these problems. Right now, the information in this book is the most complete, up-to-date information available. If you're looking for further reading material, see the reference section at the end of the book.

I'm scared to have a bowel movement. What do I do?

The first thing you should do is relax! Your fear may be your biggest enemy. It can exacerbate your problems and lead you in harmful directions. Relaxation exercises will greatly reduce your stress. Relaxation is a broad term. I use it to refer to anything we do that reduces anxiety in our daily lives. This can include reading, going to a movie, exercising, playing a game, singing, talking on the phone, or visiting a friend. Whatever works for you.

Meditation is also an excellent relaxation technique. I use it all the time. We meditate many times each day without even realizing it. Meditation is simply the process of using our brains to relax our bodies. This automatically puts our bodies in a receptive, healing state. My favorite meditation involves imagining situations I derive pleasure from. I often picture myself floating on a raft down a gentle river. Sometimes I envision this river being my thoughts. I let these thoughts flow by as I float down the river.

Another of my favorite meditations is to silently chant an important hope or wish. When I was in college, in fact, I would meditate on absorbing the information in my books or performing well on an upcoming exam. Discomfort should not be part of meditation for most people. All you need to do is find a comfortable position (whether sitting or lying down) and pick whatever form of meditation works for you.

The second thing you should do if you're afraid of having bowel movements is follow the advice I've laid out in this book. (Of course, you should check with your health practitioner to make sure this advice is correct for you!) I can summarize this advice in a few simple steps:

- Adjust your daily intake of water. If your bowel movements are too hard, drink more water. (Eight or more glasses per day is a good amount.) If they are too loose, try drinking less water.

- Increase your daily fiber intake. Of your entire diet, 70% should be vegetables (most of which contain plentiful fiber. See Chapter 9 for specific information about fibrous foods).

- If necessary, use stool softeners. These can be over-the-counter or prescription medications. Your doctor will help find the right medication for you.

I see blood in the toilet after every bowel movement. Should I be worried about cancer?

First off, call your doctor! Should you worry? Probably not. Blood in your stool is often the result of a fissure, which (as discussed in Chapter 3) is a mild to severe tear in the rectal wall. Fissures are usually not serious, and once you've regulated your bowels, fissures will heal and no longer leave blood in your stool. (Consult your doctor, however, if the condition persists. Chapter 6 on constipation will give you a great deal of information about how to heal fissures.)

If you do not suffer from constipation, but you still have blood in your stool, this is usually due to IBS (Irritable Bowel Syndrome) or polyps. In either case, consult your doctor immediately!

What can I do for the pain immediately?

Hemorrhoids and constipation can cause very different types of pain. Each type of pain involves a different solution.

Pain related to gas.

If your pain is related to gas, you should try this exercise: lie on your back with your knees up and your feet on the floor. Massage your stomach area in gentle circular motions. It's helpful to have a picture on hand of your alimentary canal, so you can massage your stomach area in the direction that your food travels. (See the diagram in Chapter 6.) After relaxing and massaging your stomach area, grab you're knees and hug them to your chest. Don't hold your breath through this exercise! Instead, breathe normally. Relax and eliminate gas as you hug your knees into your chest.

Pain related to cramps.

Sometimes your pain can be associated with intestinal cramps. These cramps may indicate a mild irritation of the intestinal lining, or—if there is blood in your stool—a more serious inflammation. The lining of your intestines is usually coated with mucus. This protects the intestines from irritation and harm. If your body produces too much acidic or alkaline digestant, the mucus lining may wear thin. This will irritate your lining and cause inflammation or swelling. It is this swelling that causes your pain. The best way to address this kind of pain is to follow the guidelines for healthy eating presented in Chapter 9.

Pain related to hemorrhoids.

A third type of pain is related to hemorrhoids. If there is no blood in your stool, yet you feel raw at your anus, most likely you have irritated the tender tissue there. This can be caused by toilet paper that is too rough or stools that are too hard. It may also occur because you are straining too much during bowel movements. First, you should make sure your toilet paper is soft. Second, you can often soothe hemorrhoidal discomfort by using creams or ointments. Third, try not to strain while having your bowel movements. (See Chapter 10 for a description of the proper way to have a bowel movement.)

I feel I have to strain to have a bowel movement. Is this bad?

There is no reason why you should have to strain to have a bowel movement. For help in relieving strain, see Chapter 6 on constipation and Chapter 9 on how to eat healthfully. If you are straining several times a day, you may be suffering from IBS. If this is the case, see your doctor immediately.

If your bowel movements are irregular and hard, you may benefit from the temporary relief that enemas and suppositories provide. Remember, though, if you increase the fluids and fiber in your diet, you will handle this problem for the long term. Enemas and suppositories can only provide temporary relief.

I have diarrhea, so how can I possibly have hemorrhoids?

Chronic diarrhea is sometimes a sign of IBS. If you have IBS, the strain of the colon cramping and contracting may cause hemorrhoids to form. Often times, hemorrhoids caused by chronic diarrhea are accompanied by pain and bleeding. This condition can be moderate to severe. Call your physician and get your condition diagnosed as soon as possible. Treatment is usually simple if the problem is identified early. Also, IBS can be prevented if you follow the advice I give in Chapters 6 and 9.

Chapter 13

One Person's Story

I have never had the misfortune of experiencing a hemorrhoidectomy. Many of you reading this book, however, may be facing just that possibility, and you may find it helpful to read the case history of a person who has had to go through this surgery. The following is my mother's story about her trials and tribulations in dealing with hemorrhoids and a hemorrhoidectomy, as told in her own words. I hope her experience will motivate you to work even harder to improve your colon health.

> I first had problems with hemorrhoids in my late twenties, after my first pregnancy. My doctor told me, "Everyone has hemorrhoids after pregnancy; they'll go away."

> I had bleeding and was in moderate discomfort for many weeks, but my hemorrhoids appeared to go away, just as my doctor had said. Whenever I was under stress, however, I noticed I would bleed and stain again. This bleeding and discomfort lasted longer and longer after each new episode.

> At 44, I developed a bladder infection and was diagnosed with uterine fibroid tumors. My doctor said the bleeding was due to a fissure and suggested suppositories as a treatment. But she didn't give me an internal examination nor did she discuss my diet with me.

Finally, at the age of 46, I visited a proctologist and was diagnosed with internal hemorrhoids. No mention was made of long term treatments. Instead, I was told to use suppositories and lotions to stop the bleeding and to alleviate my discomfort. At the same time, my gynecologist suggested I have my fibroid tumors taken out. I was given a full hysterectomy and, to my surprise, my hemorrhoids felt better after six weeks. The bleeding virtually stopped.

I still noticed that when I was under stress, I would have blood in my stool. Also, whenever I had a sigmoidoscopy I would feel some extreme pain. In 1987 I received a painful sigmoidoscopy that I believe may have injured one of my hemorrhoids. I had a great deal of discomfort, and I told my doctor about this. She gave me suppositories, but again, she didn't mention anything about my diet nor did she give me an internal exam.

Finally, in 1990 I was told by my General Practitioner to take a fiber product, yet I was not told to drink more water as well. I still did not have an internal examination until 1995.

In those five years I would have discomfort, pain, staining, and bright red blood that would sometimes fill my toilet bowl. My son, Ken, recommended that I get an internal exam. He said I shouldn't leave the doctor's office without one.

Sure enough, I was diagnosed with prolapsed hemorrhoids and was sent to a specialist. This specialist was the kindest and most thorough doctor I had ever been too. She explained that I had grade four hemorrhoids that would most likely need surgery.

At first, we tried the infrared coagulation method of treatment, and I began an extreme diet recommended by my son. This diet consisted of non-irritating fiber and mostly fruits and vegetables. To be honest, after three weeks on diet, I'd never felt better.

The discomfort and pain were mostly gone, and the bleeding had all but stopped. After three months, I went back for an exam which revealed that the grade four hemorrhoids were still present. My smaller hemorrhoids, however, had disappeared. After talking with my proctologist, I decided to have surgery. But I was not prepared for what followed.

Before I could have surgery, I had a few complications to overcome. My husband of 48 years died, and I found myself terribly depressed. I overate and was stressed about finances.

Six months before being operated on, my blood pressure was up, and I had high cholesterol. The medication I took for this made me constipated and increased my hemorrhoid problem.

Three months before the operation, my son advised me to prepare my body for the surgery. Following his advice, I went on a rigorous diet, and I began to feel better and better. I also began to meditate. Finally, my blood pressure stabilized, and I was able to go off the medication.

With the help of my kind specialist, I found the best surgeon for my surgery. My son suggested a few supplements along with a diet that prepared my body for surgery and post surgery.

I can see now just how important this preparation for my operation was. I wasn't prepared, however, for the post-operation process. After surgery, I was given a printed sheet explaining that I would be in a great deal of pain for two days. This instruction sheet also directed me to take pain killers, to get rest, to include more fiber in my diet, and to use stool softeners if I needed them. But this information didn't really convey to me all the facts.

The facts, as I experienced them, were as follows. After surgery I felt like someone had put a hot poker up me.

Every time I felt like evacuating, I was filled with fear. Because of intense swelling in my bottom area, I was at times not even able to urinate.

I had been told that after surgery it would be helpful to have someone drive me home, and later, to help me go shopping and cook my meals. Not only is it helpful, it's absolutely mandatory to have someone with you for at least five days after surgery! I was so disoriented from the drugs, there was no way I could have cared for myself.

Ken was there to administer my medications. If not for him I would have definitely over medicated myself because the pain was excruciating. All I wanted was for the pain stop so I might sleep until this whole thing was over.

Ken explained to me that the medication would constipate me, which would be counter productive to the healing process. He helped me when I needed to go to the bathroom. He also rushed me to the emergency room when I was unable urinate for almost two days.

I spent most of my waking time relaxing in a hot bath. Ken also made high fiber nutritional drinks and forced me to drink them. I had no desire to eat or drink; but if it wasn't for the soup broth and high fiber nutritional drinks, I have no doubts I would have died.

Needless to say, dying was not the worst of my alternatives. I tried to get my doctor on the phone many times to ask whether my experiences were normal; I also wanted to know what to do for my pain and lack of urinating.

Ken finally reached my doctor. After Ken explained my situation, the doctor said that I was doing a good job, but that if I didn't urinate in one more day I should be taken to the emergency room. Ken did not wait, he took me to the emergency room that evening. I was catheterized and drained of my fluid. I felt relief and this allowed me to continue the healing process.

From here on out, I basically followed nutritional instructions perfectly. I had three high fiber nutritional drinks per day and included one food at a time until I felt comfortable in my stomach and was eliminating easily and regularly.

At this point in time, my diet is simpler than it has ever been. 70% of my diet is vegetables, fruits and grains. I have about 15 to 20% proteins from eggs and fish. Sometimes chicken and very little red meat. I still make myself a high fiber drink every morning, and I find with this program I have no problems eliminating.

It has been 6 months after my surgery and not only have I prevented hemorrhoids from reappearing, I have never felt better in my life.

The Colon Health Society

All the products mentioned in this book and listed in the Resource Directory, as well as many others specific to colon health, are available at a discount through *The Colon Health Society.*

The Society also provides the following benefits to its members: the latest information on how to heal colon problems such as hemorrhoids and constipation; listings of helpful books; special discounts on products; and the best information about products available anywhere. Our approach is always both medical and naturopathic.

Whatever your needs, please feel free to write us, go to our website, or call our toll free number listed below. We will be happy to help you in any way we can.

The Colon Health Society
505 S. Beverly Drive #438
Beverly Hills, CA 90212
800-745-0791

http://www.colonhealth.com
esteem@starone.com

Visit us online!

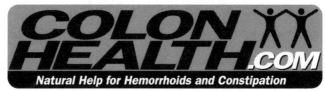

at
http://www.colonhealth.com

All the products listed in this book, as well as many others specific to colon health, are available at a discount to **Colon Health Society** members.

The **Colon Health Society**, along with our new website **"WWW.COLONHEALTH.COM"** provide the latest news, the best product information available anywhere, helpful books and special discounts to our members. Our approach is always both medical and naturopathic. And best of all - **Membership is FREE!**

Write to us at the address below, send us e.mail, visit our website, or call the toll free number listed below. Our health professionals are always ready to help!

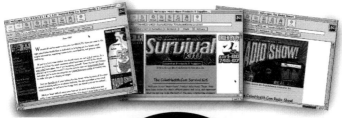

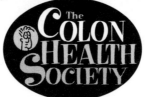

The Colon Health Society
505 S. Beverly Drive #438
Beverly Hills, CA 90212
Tel: 1.800.745.0791
Http://www.colonhealth.com
E.Mail: esteem@starone.com

Appendix A

The History of the Toilet
How the Toilet Compromises
Colon Health[3]

One of the bowel's greatest enemies in our ultramodern society is the ergonomic nightmare called the toilet. "Uncivilized" societies have always squatted. When we use the natural squatting position, our thighs directly support the abdominal wall, and this reinforces and aligns our bowels. Adopting this position can result in many significant health benefits.

The toilet first became popular in England in approximately 1850, and its use soon spread throughout the civilized world. It spread quickly because it came on the scene at the same time as plumbing, which allowed for the clean disposal of what had previously been embarrassingly stored in chamber pots or dumped into the street.

The toilet was originally designed by Joseph Bramah, a cabinetmaker, and later improved upon by Thomas Crapper, a plumber. Bramah and Crapper were not men of medicine, and neither understood the mechanical advantage that squatting afforded the body. The general public was similarly ignorant of the advantages of squatting, which explains why the toilet became popular so quickly.

It was not until the early 1900's that wise doctors—faced with a dramatically increased incidence of disease—ques-

---

[3] This appendix was written by Dr. William Welles.

tioned many modern conventions of the time, and the convention that proved most suspect was the toilet. In one book written in 1924 called *The Culture of the Abdomen*, the author quotes leading medical authorities who were outspoken about the toilet's faulty design and ensuing health consequences. The author, Frederick Hornibrook (a physical therapist), concludes the following:

> Man's natural attitude during defecation is a squatting one, such as may be observed among field workers or natives. Fashion, in the guise of the ordinary toilets, forbids the emptying of the lower bowel in the way nature intended…. It is no over statement to say that the adoption of the squatting attitude would in itself help in no small measure to remedy the greatest physical vice of the white race: constipation.

Hornibrook goes on to make this comment about the invention of the toilet: "It would have been better that the contraption had killed its inventor before he launched it under humanity's buttocks!"

Constipation, hernias, varicose veins, hemorrhoids, and appendicitis were all attributed to use of the toilet. A solution to the dilemma was offered in the form of a footstool used to elevate the feet to approximate the squatting posture. At one point this footstool became so popular that it was sold at Harrods of London.

How the Toilet Fails To Support Our Bowels
All of the undesirable consequences of using the toilet result from the simple fact that sitting and bearing down on

a toilet seat robs us of the support to our abdominal wall and colon normally afforded by squatting.

When we sit on a toilet, our thighs are not able to support the ileocecal valve as they would if we were to squat. This lack of support may compromise the mechanical dynamics of this valve. When this valve becomes compromised, there is a greater chance that fecal matter will reflux from the large intestine into the small intestine. As a result, fecal bacteria may proliferate and travel up the small intestine, to become eventually absorbed into the bloodstream. These toxins, once in the bloodstream, may cause harm to our other organs.

The phenomenon of fecal bacteria and contents entering the small intestine is so commonplace that the ileocecal valve is now being described as inherently incompetent in many modern day medical textbooks. This viewpoint, however, stands in direct opposition to what anatomists and physicians have stated.

Major symptoms of ileocecal valve dysfunction are low back and hip problems caused by the reactive weakening of muscles in the lower right quadrant of the abdomen. Other symptoms include dark circles under the eyes and an alternating consistency of stool with a tendency toward diarrhea.

Incomplete elimination of our waste can be another problem related to the use of the toilet. One physician, Dr. John Chiene, became so convinced that the toilet caused incomplete bowel movements that he actually weighed and compared the fecal mass he passed on the toilet with what he passed in a squatting position. He found that when he used the toilet, his bowel movements always weighed less, and he concluded that this was due to incomplete elimination.

The majority of all bowel problems are located in two areas of the bowel, the cecum in the lower right quadrant and the sigmoid in the lower left quadrant. These two areas are also happen to be contracted by the thighs when we use the squatting position to perform a bowel movement. When we use the toilet, we apply to pressure to these areas, which may allow fecal matter to stagnate there.

In his book *The Prevention of the Diseases Peculiar to Civilization*, Sir William Arbuthnot Lane asserts (as did Hippocrates, the father of medicine), that the standard for sound general health was one bowel movement after every meal. Dr. Lane based this opinion on a simple discovery he made. Many of the patients he operated on had a strictured area at the far end of their large intestines. This stricture seemed to "plug up" his patient's colon, thus causing constipation. He believed this stricture was caused by the use of the toilet to evacuate. When he pulled this plug, so to speak, people seemed to get well from almost everything!

Dr. Lane's method for pulling this plug was to surgically remove it, and he wrote the following about this procedure:

> Should simple measures of diet and habit fail, the freeing of the intestinal tract by operation restores its mechanics to the condition that existed in infancy. The effects are tremendous; far and away beyond what I expected. Men and woman are transformed. They become bright and happy and well. Not only do the particular

ills of which they complain disappear, but mi-
nor troubles go with them.

Unfortunately, these tremendous results were short lived. For the usual patient, the bowel would restricture precisely where it had been surgically repaired, most likely, according to Dr. Lane, because the patient continued using the toilet rather than squatting. Sir Lane explored alternatives to his surgery. He attempted to redesign the toilet, but unfortunately, he died before he could finish this project.

When World War II came along, the whole issue of the toilet's ill-conceived design was soon forgotten. In the resource directory of this book, you will find information about *The Welles Step*, a footstool which allows one to adopt a close approximation of the natural squatting position when using a toilet. This device has helped many people relieve their constipation and hemorrhoids.

Appendix B

QUICK REFERENCE SYMPTOM GUIDE

SYMPTOMS   **HELP**

**Bloated, Belly Or
Belly Bulge -** Aloe juice, Digestive enzymes*, Multi-source calcium (citrate, carbonate, oratate) with Magnesium

* 1. Betaine HCl for slow bowel movement to be taken after meals.
  2. Pancreatic Enzymes for good to fast bowel movement to be taken before meals.

**Sluggish or Slow
Irregular Bowels -** Betaine HCl (after meals), mineral enriched beverages (electrolytes) or electrolyte tablets, 32 oz. of water per day, soluble fiber, friendly intestinal bacteria such as that in acidopholis-type products/probiotics

Constipation - Betaine HCl (after meals), fiber, 32 oz. or MORE of water per day, exercise, avoid dense foods (meat, dairy, fats and peanut butter, etc.) and irritants such as chocolate, coffee, alcohol, processed sugar and white flour

Diarrhea - Soluble fiber, chlorophyll, aloe juice, acidopholis-type supplement/probiotic, electrolyte drinks or electrolyte tablets (at least 32 oz. a day)

Anal Itch - Salves & creams, aloe juice, Chlorophyll, Digestabs, soluble fiber, lots of cooked green vegetables

Hemorrhoids - Soluble fiber, electrolyte & mineral beverages, 64 oz. of water daily, avoid dense foods (meats, dairy, fats, etc.), avoid irritants (coffee, chocolate, carbonation etc.), Chlorophyll, Digestive Enzymes, Epsom Salt/mineral sitz baths, Hot & Cold devices, and may require salves & creams, Comfy Cushion

Kenneth Yasny, Ph.D. ©1997

Appendix C

Seating Cushions[4]

The purpose of most therapeutic seating cushions is either to help evenly distribute the pressure of sitting or to enhance one's positioning while sitting. Most cushions do both.

For people who are confined to a wheel chair, seating cushions are designed to distribute weight as evenly as possible so there will be no areas of concentrated pressure.

For those who have undergone rectal or pelvic surgery, or who suffer from a tailbone injury or generalized pelvic discomfort, the design of the cushion must be somewhat different. Here, the weight does not need to be evenly distributed, but rather, the sitting position must be enhanced so that the weight on some areas is eliminated (or reduced) and transferred to other areas.

The area between the legs, from roughly the pubic area in front to the tailbone in back, is called the perineum. Discomfort in this area can be brought on by wounds caused by various circumstances, including child birth, vaginal surgery, rectal surgery, or a broken tailbone. These wounds will only heal if there is proper blood flow and they are kept clean and dry.

Blood flow will not be adequate if there is too much pressure to the wounded area. Lack of blood flow will not only prevent the wound from healing, but it will also cause the

---

4 This appendix was written by Dr. Steven Goldman.

normal skin and muscle tissue to deteriorate. To understand why this is so, try a little experiment. Press your finger on the back of your hand and then let go. What do you see? You see a pale spot because you have pressed the blood out the area. What happens when you put a string or rubber band around your finger? It begins to hurt and throb because there is not enough blood flow. It would eventually die if the band were not removed.

This is just what happens when a doctor ties a baby's umbilical cord at birth. Following any sort of perineal surgery or injury, there needs to be good blood flow to speed healing and reduce pain.

It is also important for a wound to be open to air so it may "breathe," When we hold our hands in water too long, they become soft and wrinkled. We say that they are macerated. Normally, dry skin provides an effective barrier against infection. If our skin is macerated, it becomes porous and bacteria can penetrate and cause infection. It is therefore important that a wound be kept clean and dry so that it can properly heal.

Following a perineal injury, the type of seating cushion most often purchased is a donut cushion. We have all seen these at one time or another. Almost two million donut cushions are sold each year. Most are some sort of inflatable device or a ring of foam covered with a pillow case. Considering that there is almost universal agreement that these cushions are useless, it is amazingly that people buy them. There isn't one study in the scientific or medical literature to support the use of the donut cushion, yet hospitals continue to hand them out to patients following child births, hemorrhoidectomies, tailbone injuries and so on.

When you think about the design of a cushion, it is immediately apparent why it doesn't work. Because the donut is a round cushion, when you sit on it, the pressure of your body effectively creates a tourniquet around the injured area. This cuts off the two things most vital to a healing wound: blood flow and air flow. Even worse, because the donut cushion is ring-shaped like a toilet seat, it pulls the perineal area apart and puts extra strain on the injured area. Positioning the donut is also very difficult. Most of the time the injured area is not exactly in the center of the ring, but is on its edges, where all the pressure of this type of cushion is concentrated.

If the donut cushion is so untherapeutic, why is it so widely used? Firstly, it has been around a long time and is widely recognized. Secondly, it's inexpensive. In most of its various shapes and sizes, the donut cushion retails for around $20. Thirdly, and perhaps most importantly, this is the only type of cushion that has been available for people wanting relief from perineal injuries. With no other options available, people have really had no choice.

In 1986, Dr. Stephen L. Goldman realized that his clients needed an alternative to the donut cushion. This prompted him to develop a completely new type of cushion, granted a U.S. patent to cover both its design and construction. Dr. Goldman dubbed this cushion the "Comfy Cushion," and it is currently the only product available that reduces pressure to the perineum without reducing blood circulation or air flow.

It relieves most people's pelvic pain, whether from long standing pelvic discomfort or from rectal surgery, a tailbone injury, or childbirth. It transfers pressure away from painful areas to the thighs, which are in fact designed to bare this weight.   At the same time, the perineal area is gently held together to reduce stretching. The cushion feels firm at first. It is designed to gradually mold to each individual's body shape, like a new pair of shoes that become more comfortable the more they're used.

Glossary

alimentary canal: (also known as the digestive tract) is what I often refer to as "our pipes." It is the passageway through which food passes from mouth to anus, in the process of being digested and absorbed through the intestinal wall.

anthropology: the study of humans and their origins.

balanced intestinal environment: when the colon has the right amount of bacterium to allow it to function efficiently.

banding: a technique used to treat hemorrhoids that have prolapsed (as have grade three and grade four hemorrhoids). Banding entails placing a band (much like a rubber band) at the base or neck of a hemorrhoid to stop circulation. This causes the hemorrhoid to shrivel up and fall off.

injection therapy: a treatment for grades three and four hemorrhoids that is similar to the method used to remove varicose veins. In injection therapy, a saline solution is injected into the hemorrhoidal vein in order to shrink it. The disadvantage of this technique is that its uses are limited, the advantage is that the discomfort is slight.

bioflavonoids: found in fruits and plants. Such fruits and plants are loaded with antioxidant properties and are good for the repair of soft tissues (such as gums, bruises, artery walls etc.).

body message: a "voice" from the body that we "hear" through symptoms or cravings.

body wisdom: the process of the body that directs us to do what is best for us; as when we lose our hunger after a balanced meal.

cecum: the first part of the small intestine, directly below the ileocecal valve.

colitis: a form of Irritable Bowel Syndrome. Colitis can range from chronic spasms in the colon to bleeding (or ulcerative) colitis, which is quite severe.

cleansing crisis: the crisis our body goes through when we begin to eat and care for ourselves in a way that allows our body to heal itself. It is a natural, self-healing mechanism.

colorectal: pertaining to or involving the colon and rectum (as in colorectal cancer heaven forbid).

constipation: usually thought of as hardened stools or irregularity.

Crohn's disease: inflammation of the last part of the small intestine (known as the ileum). This disease can be serious enough to inhibit nutrient absorption.

cryotherapy: a treatment for grades three and four hemorrhoids. In this treatment, the hemorrhoids are frozen so that they shrink and fall off. It causes some discomfort, usually lasting from three to seven days.

dense foods: dense foods include meats and fats. I label foods as dense if they are difficult to digest and are heavier than fruits, vegetables and carbohydrates.

diverticulitus: inflammation of diverticula, which are sac-like herniations through the colon's muscular wall. Diverticulitus is characterized by abdominal pain, fever, and changes in bowel movements, such as diarrhea.

disease state: the condition of having a diagnosable health problem.

fats: see oils.

fiber: the part of our food which is indigestible. Fiber helps us by carrying our wastes out of the body.

fissures: tears in the rectal lining (or sometimes on a hemorrhoid) that will bleed.

food categories: a way of grouping foods according to their chemical molecular structure. This is done because foods with different molecular structures require different enzymes in order to be broken down during digestion. The general food categories are simple carbohydrates, complex carbohydrates, proteins, fats, oils, and dairy products.

grades of hemorrhoids: hemorrhoids are graded in severity from grade one (which is the least severe) to grade four (which is the most severe).

hemorrhoidectomy: the surgical removal of hemorrhoids.

hemorrhoids: veins in the rectum. We usually assume that hemorrhoids protrude from the intestinal wall, though technically speaking, this is not necessarily the case.

hominid: a primate from whom modern man is believed to have evolved.

IBS: Irritable Bowel Syndrome. This is an umbrella term used to describe conditions ranging from chronic diarrhea to ulcerative colitis.

ileocecal valve: a valve located at the end of the small intestine, before the colon.

infrared coagulation: a treatment which shows promising results for addressing grade one, grade two, and grade three hemorrhoids. It involves exposing hemorrhoids to infrared light, which hopefully causes them to retreat back into the intestinal lining where they belong. It is a relatively non-invasive technique and only causes a minimum of discomfort (usually lasting a couple days).

large intestine: the colon.

legumes: foods from the plant family Leguminosae. Common examples are beans, peas, peanuts, alfalfa, clover, indigo, and lentil.

lymph: a fluid in the blood that helps clean up the "gunk" left behind by the immune system's battles with invasive organisms.

oils: I like to make a distinction between fats and oils. I consider fats to come from meat, dairy, and fried foods. These fats are usually the kind that can raise cholesterol levels. (They are often referred to as saturated fats.) Oils, unlike fats, remain liquid at room temperature and are usually unsaturated.

perineum: the perineum, also known as the pelvic floor, is the space between the anus and genitals.

peristalsis: the progressive wave of contraction and relaxation of a muscular system, especially the alimentary canal, by which the contents (foods) are pushed through the system (pipes).

physiognomy: facial features.

pilates: a sophisticated method of exercising all muscle groups.

plexus: a network of nerves or blood vessels (as in the hemorrhoidal plexus in the anus).

prolapse: when an organ (such as hemorrhoidal veins) fall or slips out of place.

radiating pain: pain that spreads out or travels from its point of origin to another spot of the body, as in the case of a heart attack (in which pain travels from the chest down the left arm) or gas (in which pain in the colon can radiate to the ribs).

reflux: a flowing back.

sigmoid: the last part of the colon. It has an 's' curve to it.

sigmoidoscopy: a tube with a camera and tools at its end that is sent up the sigmoid.

sitz bath: a soothing bath with healing minerals added.

sphincter: any muscle that has the ability to tightly close or open (for example, the anus).

stomach: a pouch-like jumble of strong muscles (the size of our fist) that churns up food in preparation for digestion. It is located at the top of our alimentary canal.

stool: our waste or excrement (also known as poop, turd, ca ca, etc.).

stool softeners: these are caplets, pearles, suppositories and various other ointments and creams that can be used to soften stool. They are used to counter, and sometimes treat, constipation. Most stool softeners are liquid filled pearles, suggested to add "slip" to the stool.

suppositories: bullet shaped anal inserts that can soothe our bowels, can stimulate a bowel movement, and can help reduce swelling of the anus.

succanat: a natural, unbleached sugar that comes from sugar cane.

thrombosis: a blood clot.

thrombosed hemorrhoid: a hemorrhoid that has formed a clot.

transit time: the time it takes for food to go through our entire alimentary canal.

vegan: a vegan is one who eats no animal products whatsoever; this includes no milk, cheese, eggs, or dairy products.

vegetarian: one who eats no meats, yet may eat dairy and eggs.

yoga: a balanced method of exercise. There are many schools of yoga. Some are mild; others are intensely active.

Resource Directory

4Health, Inc.

Nature's Secret products are formulated by Lindsey Duncan, CN, founder and head nutritionist of the well respected Home Nutrition Clinic in Santa Monica, California, and founder and CEO of 4Health, Inc., a leading supplier of four brands of herbal and nutritional supplements. After years of research and helping more than 10,000 people attain better health, Lindsey is convinced that internal cleansing is the first step to health. We at *4Health, Inc.* recommend that the three Nature's Secret internal cleansing products - **Ultimate Cleanse** ™, **Ultimate Fiber** ™, and **Ultimate Oil** ™ - be taken together as a program to achieve optimum results. In addition, Super Cleanse ™, is recommended for individuals who have a more sluggish colon and need an extra *"jump start"* to initiate their internal cleansing program.

Ultimate Cleanse is a two part, internal body cleansing formula that helps your body flush out toxins by targeting and supporting five channels of elimination (bowel, skin, kidneys, lungs, and lymphatic system)

Ultimate Fiber contains sources of soluble *and* insoluble fiber that sweep and tone the intestines *gently*, without swelling or gelling like most other fiber products.

Ultimate Oil contains a unique blend of cold pressed oils containing essential fatty acids which are essential to the healthy functioning of every organ, tissue and cell in your body. Taken in easy-to-swallow capsules, it will soothe and lubricate your entire digestive and elimination systems.

Super Cleanse is an extra-strength bowel cleansing formula designed to promote 2 to 3 good bowel movements every day, for individuals with a more sluggish colon, who do not get the desired results with Ultimate Cleanse, Ultimate Fiber, and Ultimate Oil.

For more information on Nature's Secret products or internal cleansing, call 1-800-29 SECRET weekdays 7:00 am to 5:30 PM (MST).

Agape Health Products

"Take the First Step to Better Health"

Perfect 7 is a natural, gentle, bulk forming, water-soluble fiber powder, used for the relief of occasional constipation and irregularity. This formula has been in use for over 20 years. Perfect 7 can help relieve constipation and help establish regularity which can be an important contribution to overall health.

Herbal Laxative Tablets are a safe, natural way to encourage elimination. They are an aid in the relief of occasional constipation and associated symptoms. Gentle and effective, generally produces comfortable elimination within 8 hours or overnight.

Herbal Laxative Tea combination assists the body in mild cleansing and detoxification. It's mild flavor and gentle action make it a desirable and comforting aid in the relief of constipation and irregularity. One cup in the morning and one cup at night is beneficial.

Look for all these fine products at a health food store in your neighborhood.

Age In Reverse

LIVING ON EARTH IN HARMONY WITH GRAVITY

Relaxing your body on the *BODYSLANT* is a perfectly natural way to reverse the downward pull of gravity on your face, neck, shoulders, chest, back, organs, hips, legs and feet.

Indeed, the concept and practice of counteracting gravity's force on the human body is an ancient and proven rejuvenating technique. Lying on the modern BODYSLANT, moreover, is as safe and easy as lying on a bed.

Lying on a *BODYSLANT* readily improves the circulation of blood to your increasing the flow of blood and oxygen to your head instantly washes away tension and headaches. It's also valuable to your vision, hearing, scalp, complexion and memory.

THE NEW SLANT FOR UPRIGHT PEOPLE

As an abiding heads-up person (that is, someone who sits and stands all day, then sleeps with their head on top of a pillow all night) your body will definitely feel inclined on taking a *TEN-MINUTE BODYSLANT BREAK.*

Simply stretching out your body on the *BODYSLANT* (with your head lower than your heart - and your feet higher than your heart) is a comfortable and enjoyable way to upgrade your youth and vitality.

The benefits of overturning gravity's pull on your mind and body, with the aid of *BODYSLANT*, are immediate and unmistakable. Your posture will be more erect. Your abdomen will be visibly flatter. You'll experience a wonderful new lightness in your every movement.

The feeling of truly enhancing your mental and physical well-being, while resting on the *BODYSLANT*, will obviously go to your head.

For more information, please call: 714-631-2241

Aloe Flex Products, Inc.

Hemorrhoid Lotion. This is the most effective, all natural method to relieve the discomfort of hemorrhoids, both internal and external. It is cooling, soothing and relieves inflammation and swelling. Comprised of 89% Aloe Vera. Prevents recurrence. FDA approved to sell at all drug and health food stores.

Perianal Lotion. Developed for the treatment of hemorrhoids as a way to wash and cleanse the affected area while soothing the area at the same time. Aloe Flex processes only pure aloe vera including the entire leaf, into a fine line of health products. Patient approved and doctor tested, no side effects and above all, they work!

Write or call for free information. You'll be glad you did. 800-231-0839. Write us at PO Box 1347 Dickinson, TX 77539

BHI - Biological Homeopathic Industries

There are many ways of treating the painful symptoms of constipation and hemorrhoids. Heel/BHI is a manufacturer of complex homeopathic medicines with safe and natural remedies for effective relief of these common complaints. Heel/BHI offers tablets, suppositories, and ointments, for a wide variety of treatment options.

BHI Constipation tablets provide temporary relief of constipation due to changes in diet, improper nutrition, or inadequate exercise. *BHI Constipation* is also effective for constipation accompanying stomach and abdominal pains.

To many people, the burning and itching associated with hemorrhoids are the worst aspects of this condition. *BHI Hemorrhoid* is a remedy available both in tablets and suppositories. In either form, *BHI Hemorrhoid* reduces the swollen tissue and accompanying soreness.

BHI Paeonia ointment, made from the peony flower, provides soothing relief from the incessant itching. *BHI Paeonia* is a perfect complement to *BHI Hemorrhoid* suppositories and tablets, for complete relief.

For more information about these natural medicines for constipation and hemorrhoids, visit your local health food store today.

Camilla Corporation

Why the *Comfy Cushion*? The Comfy Cushion was developed by Dr. Steven Goldman, a practicing Colon & Rectal Surgeon, to fill the needs of his patients. Following rectal or pelvic surgery, patients would purchase a donut cushion to help relieve pressure to sensitive areas. They would then comment that not only does the donut not help them, but in fact makes them worse. When you think about it, this makes perfect sense. A ring is like a toilet seat which is designed to separate the buttocks which puts tension on sore areas. At the time, there was no alternative on the market. As a result, he started on the development of the Comfy Cushion.

The basic concept was a cushion which would both relieve pressure from sore and tender areas and not separate the buttocks. During the seven plus years of development, he would produce prototypes which were distributed to patients, and subsequent models were modified based on their comments and feedback. In essence, the *Comfy Cushion* was designed by the patients who needed it and used it.

The current *Comfy Cushion* is the result of these efforts, and is the only cushion on the market that provides satisfactory relief following any sort of pelvic surgery. Patients with hemorrhoidal problems, painful tailbones and generalized pelvic discomfort are helped immeasurably.

For more information call: 800-893-2263

Enzymatic Therapy

A leader in the natural health industry, produces more than 200 effective natural medicines and nutritional supplements, and distributes them worldwide. Our product line includes a wide variety of vitamins, minerals, standardized herbal extracts, homeopathic medicines, and natural OTC products.

Hemorrhoid Remedy - This oral homeopathic medicine relieves the pain, itching, burning, tenderness, and swelling of hemorrhoids - without side effects or toxicity! In contrast, some topical hemorrhoid products cause inflammation and burning.

Hem-Tone - The vascular system, including the veins in and around the rectum, needs nutritional support. This is especially important for people who suffer from constipation. Hem-Tone™ supports the veins in that area with nutrients such as vitamins E, calcium lactate, phosphorous, and vitamin B12.

VariCare - Many people are concerned about painful veins in their legs and around the rectum. VariCare provides standardized herbal extracts such as butchers broom horse chestnut, and Gotu kola Phytosome® that nutritionally support proper circulation and healthy veins.

Look for all these fine products at a health food store in your neighborhood. Questions? - Call Enzymatic Therapy at 1-800-783-2286.

Hepp Industries

CLEN-ZONE - The First Anal Cleansing Appliance

The greatest advance in bathroom habits since indoor plumbing!

ClenZone, the Hygiene Machine...A MUST FOR HEMMORRHOID SUFFERERS. Practically a Liquid Toilet Tissue. Easily installed on any commode without costly plumbing. It is no longer necessary to get clean with dry toilet tissue after performing a bodily function. ClenZone's gentle, controlled super narrow jet stream washes so thoroughly without splashing and soaking that you only use a few toilet tissues to pat dry.

Aside from the benefits of daily intimate cleansing, the soothing waters of the *ClenZone Hygiene Machine* relieve the discomforts of hemorrhoids, rashes, itching... is a godsend after childbirth, after surgery, during menstruation.

Protects against infections. And much, much more. With an exclusive metering attachment you can mix warm water with medicated or cleansing solutions. It's an essential in every family. For men, women and children.

The ClenZone Hygiene Machine is simply a small, ingenious plastic attachment anyone can permanently install on any commode. Needs no electricity. No plumbing. ClenZone attaches to any bathroom sink with a handsome chrome-plated diverter valve with built-in no-splash aerator.

HEPP Industries, Inc., TEL: 516-253-3342 FAX: 516-253-0218

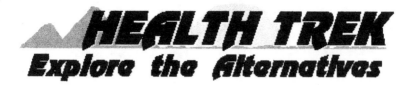

*Over 500 **all natural** homeopathic & herbal products...*
including these Hemorrhoid remedies!

HEMORRHOID GEL

Homeopathic gel relieves pain and itching of hemorrhoids. Helps to shrink swelling. *2 oz. gel.*

LIVER GALL BLADDER EXTRA

Homeopathic for the temporary relief of flatulence, constipation, belching, abdominal discomfort, dysfunction, liver, gall bladder, hemorrhoids and cholesterol. *1 fl. oz.*

INDIGESTION

Homeopathic liquid for temporary relief of digestion problems associated with hemorrhoids. *1 fl. oz.*

HEMORRHOID COMP

Herbal liquid for symptomatic relief of hemorrhoids. *1 fl. oz.*

All prices in U.S. Dollars.

Phone or FAX orders to: 800-756-0871 or 712-647-2413

WE ACCEPT
MASTERCARD
& VISA

More information on
hemorrhoids at
our website
www.healthtrek.com

Herbal Comfort Products

Ancient Wisdom. Modern-day Relief.

Remedy H is a Swiss product for treating hemorrhoids based on an ancient Chinese formula that has been used for over 3,000 years. *Remedy H* effectively treats hemorrhoids that are most commonly linked to postnatal stress, prolonged constipation, long periods of sitting, improper diet, lack of exercise, sedentary lifestyle or heavy lifting.

It offers relief of hemorrhoids and their symptoms, including swelling, itching, bleeding, pain, burning and prolapsed rectum. A change in diet is often recommended for those suffering with hemorrhoids. This is a great long term solution, however most hemorrhoid sufferers need fast relief. Remedy H contains the perfect combination of herbs to quickly reduce the pain and lengthen the time between episodes and their severity.

For more information, please call Herbal Comfort Products Ltd. Toll Free at: 1-888-437-2259 or 604-730-1462, or visit our web site at: www.herbalcomfort.bc.ca

Jungle Packaging

Uña *de gato* or *Cat's claw herb* (Uncaria tomentosa) comes exclusively from the highlands of the Peruvian rain forest. It is a giant, woody vine that grows to heights of more than 100 feet. The name comes from the thorns found on the vine that closely resemble the claws of a cat.

Researchers say it is an immune system and metabolic tonifying herb of the highest order - equal, if not superior in some functions, to the world's foremost tonic herbs. They also call it the *"Opener of the Way"* for its remarkable ability to cleanse the intestinal tract, clearing the way so specific nutrients can do their job. For hundreds - if not thousands of years the Ashaninka Indians of Peru have used it for a wide variety of health concerns involving the immune and digestive systems.

Traditionally, both the bark and root of the vine have been used in herbal preparations. However, to maintain the delicate ecological balance of the rain forest, only the inner bark of the vine is used. As long as the root remains intact, it will naturally replenish itself. Moreover, the bark contains all the active constituents of the plant.

Scientists have isolated six alkaloids from the **uña de gato** vine. Research shows that four of these alkaloids have a pronounced enhancement effect on the ability of white blood cells and macrophages to attack, engulf and digest harmful microorganisms, foreign matter and debris.

The presence of these many alkaloids in Cat's Claw help to modify conditions in the digestive tract. It is also an excellent anti-inflammatory and has the ability to balance and modify the pH in the colon. It's strong influence in enhancing our digestive capabilities improves constipation and helps rid the body of hemorrhoids.

For more information call: 800-345-1581

A REVOLUTIONARY NEW PRODUCT

"This is the finest product in the category of tissue products that I have ever seen. I shall be recommending it to all my patients who suffer from hemorrhoids, rectal infections, and other post-traumatic conditions from surgery."

– L. Peter Fielding, M.D., F.R.C.S., F.A.C.S.,
Chief of Surgery, The Genessee Hospital
Professor of Surgery, University of Rochester School of Medicine

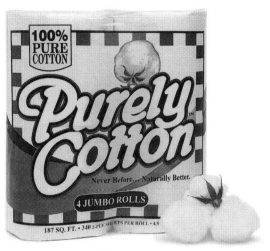

Naturally better for sensitive skin.

Purely Cotton™ is the only 100% pure cotton bathroom tissue. Doctor recommended for people with hemorrhoids.

Unlike ordinary toilet paper which is made from wood pulp and chemicals, Purely Cotton is the only premium bathroom tissue made from 100% pure cotton.

- No harsh wood-related chemicals
- Naturally soft and hypo-allergenic
- Free of inks, dyes, and perfumes
- Biodegradable and septic-safe
- Made from cotton—an environmentally-friendly, renewable resource

Now available at selected supermarkets and drugstores.
Please call 1-800-372-SOFT for the store in your area.

PUT HEMORRHOIDS AND CONSTIPATION BEHIND YOU

Lūbidet ®

TOILET ATTACHMENT: Water cleansing and warm air drying are gentle and effective. Dry wiping is traumatic. The natural wash soothes **HEMORRHOIDS** and relieves **CONSTIPATION**. Optimum comfort is achieved by using before and during a bowel movement. This lubricates the anus and relaxes the sphincter muscle.

"Hemorrhoid pain and bleeding have gone from instantly reduced to absent in a few months. No surgeon would ever wipe a dry gauze sponge across a dilated, inflamed vessel in a futile attempt to clean it. The proper maneuver is irrigation and suction. The **Lubidet** *replicates this action."* **Dr. Judd Goodman.**

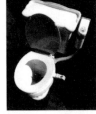

National 1st Place Winner!

AMERICAN SOCIETY ON AGING

1993

AWARD
Outstanding Product Design for Mature Consumers

FREE brochure:

Lubidet U S A Inc
1980 S Quebec St Suite 4
Denver CO 80231-3234

800-582-4338

Medi-Life

"MediLife creates and markets consumer self care software and interactive online resources for a lifetime of better health. MediLife's line of Windows-based programs simplify the management of one's health.

Balance PC Diabetes Software, enables people with diabetes to better understand, monitor, and manage their personal treatment plans. This all-inclusive program allows you to work with your health care providers to personalize your treatment plan for tighter blood glucose control.

Lighten Up, is an easy-to-use product for combining better nutrition and regular exercise into a personal weight loss plan. The program can customize this proven combination for weight loss to your schedule, your favorite foods and your favorite exercises. With 16,000 foods and hundreds of exercises in front of you, it is easy to plan healthful meals and exercise in the *Smart Health Calendar.* Set nutrient goals, analyze your meals, and decide which exercise works best for you."

For more information call toll free: 888-656-5656

Molecular Biologics, Inc.

Is one of our best resources. They produce some of the highest quality supplements and homeopathic formulas for professionals using nature's "nutriceuticals" in alternative healthcare. MBI says their potency and consistency are guaranteed by using the highest quality USP grade pharmaceutical raw materials, proprietary techniques of manufacturing unique formulas and an extremely high-tech laboratory for quality control. A great deal of science-based knowledge and clinical experience are needed to produce formulas that really work. MBI products have over ten years of clinical use and their excellent performance makes them some of the best therapeutic products available.

STONEROOT COMPLEX is the primary product, and contains a balance of several herbs for getting rid of that nasty backpressure from the liver. The balance of Stone Root, Milk Thistle, White Oak Bark, Vitamin E, Zinc, plus other herbs that work particularly well with each other, makes this a very powerful biochemical product.

MB13 HEMORRHOIDAL DROPS is a homeopathic combination formula that is specific for the symptoms of hemorrhoids. It is very safe. The debate about homeopathic products is eliminated because they either work, or they don't, but it is sure that they do no harm. This product is supposed to reduce hemorrhoidal symptoms while assisting the tissue to detoxify as well.

BIO MUCIL is a mucilloid which is very effective in both the breakdown and elimination of rotten stuff which has, over time, built up in your guts. We all have this problem. The herbs in this formula have been time-tested over 50 years. Besides cleansing, the detoxifying effects are a big help against pathogens (Yikes!). The lactalbumin provides a happy environment for our beneficial bacteria - those helpful little guys that bust up our food — to grow naturally.

BIODOPHILUS is a combination of lactobacillus acidophilus and bifidus — these boys are both bacterium, beneficial for helping to keep our digestive tract and large intestine a healthy and happy home. Any intestinal cleansing program must have a good probiotic product. This one is our best choice for maintaining good intestinal flora.

MILK THISTLE - Ours is a combination of several herbs which have a purgative effect on the liver tissue and a purifying result on both the liver and the gallbladder. Since the liver is one of the more important cleansing organs, it is very important to clean the filters a couple times per year so both organs can do their jobs.

HEPAPURG is a homeopathic combination formula which assists in liver/systemic detoxification and provides healthy energy for liver support. This product is gentle but very effective when used with the other products. Homeopathic products provide an inherent energy — which can be called "natural harmonics" — unlike biochemical energy. It is the natural harmonics which can greatly assist in the healing process.

For more information call: 800-327-4104

Nature's Path, Inc.

FLORA-LYTE ™: Five Strain Acidophilus in a Base of Electrolytes - In reestablishing healthy intestinal flora, the focus needs to be on replenishing and supporting beneficial bacteria as opposed to waging war on bacteria which upset health. To maintain and protect health, a high broad-spectrum acidophilus supplement and electrolytes should be at the top of everyone's shopping list.

LIQUID CRYSTALLOID MINERALS: Trace-Lyte™ is a true crystalloid (smallest form in nature) electrolyte formula that helps maintain the body's primary big-oxidation process. It raises the Osmotic Pressure of the cell walls, strengthening them! It changes back the pH of the cell to its healthy state. This process is generally referred to as homeostasis (electrolyte balance). High absorption is achieved due to its crystalloid structure. Some doctors have even said it acts like 'chelation' in a bottle! Unlike most earth-type liquid minerals, there is no heavy metal contaminates whatsoever. NATURE'S PATH, INC. PO Box 7862, Venice FL 34287-7862 (800)-326-5772, (941)-426-3375

Pilex

Ayurvedic herbal remedies have been used for thousands of years. We now offer an all natural herbal composition which quickly relieves the symptoms related to both internal and external hemorrhoids.

Our unique patented product in capsule form taken orally for seven days (one per day) will provide the relief necessary to stop the pain, bleeding, itching and discomfort from hemorrhoids. Our product is both Doctor tested and Doctor recommended with no side effects when used as directed. If you are searching for relief, try a wonderful alternative to conventional hemorrhoidal treatments. Pilex contains no narcotics, sugar, salt or preservatives and is only comprised of natural plant ingredients.

While legally we are not permitted to make specific claims, in a very high number of cases, we have seen dramatic improvement in only seven days, with noticeable relief from pain beginning after only a few days on the product. Testimonials and more information is available from us directly, or you may access us on the internet at http://www.hemorrhoid.com or phone us at 1-800-PILEX95.

Proper Nutrition, Inc.

Our practitioners report very effective results in using *Seacure* to relieve chronic constipation. Additionally, many patients notice significant improvement in their hemorrhoids due to the anti-inflammation and tissue repair benefits of our product.

Seacure is a whole food product made from fish. What makes Seacure unique is our special biological process which gently breaks down the protein to amino acids and small chain peptides. The doctors that use Seacure in their practice call it the most quickly absorbed and easily assimilated protein product they have ever seen. Why is this important? Because so many digestive tract problems, from indigestion and heartburn to constipation, are related to the body's inability to properly digest and absorb protein.

With *Seacure,* you give the body the critical building blocks it needs to effect repair. As many doctors tell us "a little bit of the right thing that is actually absorbed and assimilated, makes all the difference in the world".

Satisfaction guaranteed! To order or request additional information call 1-800-247-5656.

Raw Materials

*Living Food - An Organically Grown
Superfood Made with Sprouted Grains and
Seeds Harvested at the Peak of Enzyme Activity*

Living food is a balanced combination of whole foods designed to be blended into a variety of convenient, nourishing, high energy recipes. You can depend on a quick boost from Living Food when there is no time for healthy cooking or when certified organic foods are not available.

It is the only food of its type providing such a complete array of homegrown certified organic ingredients in a technologically advanced synergistic formula. when you use it, the results will speak for themselves.

Why use living food?

We have designed this combination of whole foods for those needing assistance in their transition to a better diet including many who have made already upgrades and now seek an even higher level of vitality - moving away from animal products and towards whole vegetarian foods.

What are the benefits of Living Food?

You can expect more energy and less hunger and many healing benefits throughout your body.

For more information call: 800-310-0729

The Walking Center

Are you tired of exercise equipment that you've stopped using because it hurts your body, or fails to achieve the results you wanted?

The Walking Center has been selling quality exercise equipment for the last ten years and we specialize in exercise for colon health. We feature the most technologically advanced equipment available today which is both biomechanically and ergonomically correct. Everything we recommend is designed to be safe, comfortable and efficient.

We can provide you with equipment anywhere in the United States or we will refer you to someone in your area. If you have any questions about exercise for colon health, exercise in general, or want information about any piece of equipment you might see, please call us.

For more information call: 310-275-9255

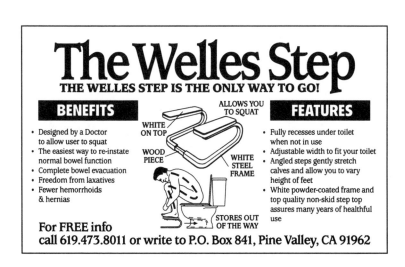

The Welles Step

THE WELLES STEP IS THE ONLY WAY TO GO!

BENEFITS

- Designed by a Doctor to allow user to squat
- The easiest way to re-instate normal bowel function
- Complete bowel evacuation
- Freedom from laxatives
- Fewer hemorrhoids & hernias

ALLOWS YOU TO SQUAT

WHITE ON TOP

WOOD PIECE

WHITE STEEL FRAME

STORES OUT OF THE WAY

FEATURES

- Fully recesses under toilet when not in use
- Adjustable width to fit your toilet
- Angled steps gently stretch calves and allow you to vary height of feet
- White powder-coated frame and top quality non-skid step top assures many years of healthful use

For FREE info call 619.473.8011 or write to P.O. Box 841, Pine Valley, CA 91962

Trace Minerals Research

Twenty five years ago, our founder, Hartley Anderson, understood the human body's need for the full spectrum of trace minerals. Today, Trace Minerals Research combines the natural balance of minerals and trace minerals with vitamins, herbs, enzymes and other nutrients to create a full line of the best products available today.

The most powerful trace minerals formula yet.

Low sodium ConcenTrace ™ Trace Mineral Drops (or tablets) are the most powerful natural health mineral supplements in the world.

It's impossible to underestimate the importance of minerals and trace minerals for the human body. They are the catalysts for all the vitamins and other nutrients your body uses for developing and maintaining good health. Using ConcenTrace ™ every day will help conduct and generate your body's entire electrical system. You'll have more energy and will generally feel better.

Cleanse your body and start feeling more healthy.

The Complete Cleansing and Anti-Toxin System is a great way to begin a health program. It works in two stages just as the body's own cleansing and anti-toxin system works in two parts.

Part one, a combination of herbs and trace minerals, helps the body filter out the toxins and waste products. Part two gently sweeps and cleanses the bowel. Fiber allows for a thorough cleanse without the discomfort of diarrhea. Best of all, it's completely natural, so you can cleanse your body without interrupting your lifestyle.

Trace Minerals Research. Family owned and operated for 25 years. If you have questions about any of these products, one of our customer service representatives will gladly help. Call us toll-free during regular business hours at 1-800-759-6993, ext. 332.

Wakunaga of America

Since the development of *Kyolic®* almost four decades ago, more research has been done on this Aged Garlic Extract™ than on all other garlic supplements combined. *Kyolic* is also covered by more than a dozen patents and patents pending worldwide. *Kyolic* is aged to bring out safer, more valuable and effective antioxidant components than fresh raw garlic. The research on *Kyolic* covers liver protection, breast, prostate and bladder cancer, AIDS, pollution, chelator of heavy metals such as mercury, lead etc., promotes the growth of friendly bacteria. The science of *Kyolic* has reached into the field of cardiovascular health with excellent research on high blood pressure, lowering cholesterol and the prevention of plaque buildup. *Kyolic* is truly odorless as well as sociable and comes in liquid, capsule and tablet forms.

Kyo•Green® is a powdered drink mix made from young barley and wheat grass, brown rice, chlorella and kelp. This combination provides you with a daily balanced amount of vitamins, minerals, enzymes, amino acids and is a great source of fiber. This is one green that really tastes great, mixes instantly and enhances the flavor of your favorite juices. *Kyo•Green* is a good natural source of chlorophyll, minerals (it is particularly high in calcium, magnesium and potassium too) vitamins and enzymes which are needed for proper metabolism. *Kyo•Green* is a rich source of antioxidant enzymes which slow down the aging process and control progression of degenerative diseases. *Kyo•Green* is a powerhouse of nutrients that alkalize and energize. *Kyo•Green* is a potent stimulator of the immune system.

The fountain of youth lies within the intestinal tract. No wonder the **British Medical Journal** said "Death begins in the colon." Antibiotics, a high meat diet, alcohol, birth control pills and stress can all upset the delicate balance of intestinal flora which is essential to achieve maximum colon health. Our colon health depends primarily on three factors; (1) existence of a slightly acidic pH, (2) maintenance of a predominantly acidophilus colon flora and, (3) regular elimination. There are two high quality products on the market that meet the above three requirements which can be used daily to insure optimum colon health. They are *Probiata®* and *Kyo•Dophilus.®* Both are sugar, yeast and dairy free, suitable for all ages and never require refrigeration which makes them ideal for daily use or travel. Both are unique because the strains of each are indigenous to the human body and therefore will colonize in the colon.

If taken two (2) hours after antibiotics, *Probiata* and *Kyo•Dophilus* are capable of preventing vaginal yeast infections. The advantages of *Probiata* and *Kyo•Dophilus* are the following: (1) they populate the colon with friendly bacteria which can inhibit the growth of harmful bacteria, viruses and toxins, (2) they may decrease the production of toxic and cancer causing compounds produced in the intestinal tract, (3) they have a cholesterol lowering effect, (4) they have a positive effect on keeping the liver functioning properly and, (5) they alleviate diarrhea, constipation, gas, bloating, poor digestion and yeast related problems.

Probiata and *Kyo•Dophilus* can play a role in estrogen metabolism by breaking down estrogen into more friendly compounds. Thus, lowering the risk to a women's health.

Probiata is available in tablet form and can be purchased only in the Mass Market and Drug Stores (for a free sample, please call 800.688.3933). *Kyo•Dophilus* is available in capsule and chewable tablet form and is available only in Health Food Stores and *Kyolic* Aged Garlic Extract is also available at your local Health Food Store (for free samples please call 800.825.7888).

Zewa Medical Systems

HOME THERAPY FOR HEMORRHOIDS?

Zewa Medical Systems has developed a unique treatment, especially for home and self-applied therapy. For this device, they received a medal at Geneve (biggest, most important invention congress in the world).

HOW THIS TREATMENT WORKS:

The therapy device is a unit controlled by a processor which heats a temperature-adjustable thermal element sealed in a rectal probe. This rectal probe, which is the shape of an elongated suppository, is introduced into the anal canal and set at a temperature which is ideal and comfortable for the patient (99° - 113° Fahrenheit). The probe radiates pulsating heat waves for 20 minute periods at the desired temperature. Application is simple, easy and perfectly hygienic. After 20 minutes the device automatically shuts down, followed by an electronic sound. This will allow the patient to know he/she is finished the treatment.

Zewa introduces three devices. The ecoversion, the smallest device, allows the patient to choose the desired temperature with a simple indicated switch on the scale. The more expensive device works with a microprocessor where the temperature chosen, temperature working, and the time lapse appears on the digital display. These two devices with a charge battery pack. The third device, on the other hand, is the doctor's version, has the same features as the microprocessor, however, the power is supplied by a security transformer on the device. This device can be used all day.

Clinical studies were made on the test results of 107 patients at the University Hospital in Zurich, Switzerland, that over 78% continued to have complete absence of ailment after 1 entire year.

Dr. Peter Buchman, Chief of Surgery, Professor of Proctology, author of several major studies on hemorrhoids, recommends usage of this device 1 - 2 times a day for a 20 minute period. Duration of therapy is 1 - 4 weeks.

You now have the opportunity to soothe your hemorrhoids with the difference of convenient home therapy in a relaxing and comfortable way.

ZEWA Inc. Medical Technology, 848 Brickell Ave., Suite #605 Miami, Florida 33131.

Tel: (305) 374-1118 Contact: Mr. Kurt Zeindler

References

Airola, P. (1977). *Hypoglycemia: A better approach.* Phoenix, AZ: Health Plus.

Airola, P. (1980). *How to keep slim, healthy, and young with juice fasting.* Phoenix, AZ: Health Plus.

Atkins, R. (1981). *Dr. Atkins' nutrition breakthrough.* New York: Bantam Books.

Asimov, Isaac. (1954). *The Chemicals of Life.* New York, New York: Signet Books.

Baldwin, E. (1972). *The nature of biochemistry.* Cambridge, Great Britain: Cambridge University Press.

Ballentine, R. (1982). *Diet and nutrition: A wholistic approach.* Honesdale, PA: The Himalayan International Institute.

Bieler, H. (1973). *Food is your best medicine.* New York: Vintage Books.

Bland, J. (1995). *Vitamin C: The future is now.* New Canaan, CT: Keats.

Cerra, F. (1984). *Pocket manual of surgical nutrition.* Princeton: The C. V. Mosby Company.

Chopra, D. (1993). *Ageless body, timeless mind : The quantum alternative to growing old.* New York: Harmony Books.

Christopher, J. (1976). *Dr. Christopher talks on rejuvenation through elimination.* Provo, UT: Self-published.

Cohen, S. (1969). *The drug dilemma.* New York: McGraw Hill.

Cousins, N. (1981). *Anatomy of an illness.* New York: Bantam Books.

Davis, A. (1965). *Let's get well.* New York: Harcourt, Brace & World.

Diamond, H., & Diamond, M. (1985). *Fit for life.* New York: Warner Books.

Diamond, H., & Diamond, M. (1987). *Living health.* New York: Warner Books.

Dufty, W. (1980). *You are all sanpaku.* Ontario, Canada: Citadel Press.

Editorial Committee of the Nutrition Foundation. (1976). *Present knowledge in nutrition.* New York: The Nutrition Foundation.

Ehret, A. (1972). *Professor Arnold Ehret's mucusless diet healing system.* Beaumont, CA: Ehret Literature Publishing. (Original work published 1922).

Esser, W. (1983). *Dictionary of natural foods.* Bridgeport, CT: Natural Hygiene Press.

Ewald, E. B. (1978). *Recipes for a small planet.* New York: Balantine Books.

Henderson, J. (1984). *Run farther run faster.* New York: McMillan Publishing.

Hoffer, A., & Walker, M. (1978). *Orthomolecular nutrition.* New Canaan, CT: Keats Publishing.

Hornibrook, F. A. (1924). *The culture of the abdomen.* New York: W. Wood & Co.

Housman, P., & Hurley, J. B. (1989). *The healing foods.* Emmaus, PA: Rodale Press.

Howell, E. (1985). *Enzyme nutrition: The food enzyme concept.* Wayne, NJ: Avery Publishing.

Insel, P., & Roth, W. (1979). *Core concepts in health.* Palo Alto, CA: Mayfield Publishing.

Jensen, B. (1979). *Nature has a remedy.* Escondido, CA: Bernard Jensen International.

Jensen, B. (1981). *Tissue cleansing through bowel management.* Escondido, CA: Bernard Jensen International.

Jensen, B. (1983). *Chemistry of man.* Escondido, CA: Bernard Jensen International.

Jensen, B. (1988). *Beyond basic health.* Wayne, NJ: Avery Publishing Group.

Jensen, B. (1988). *Rejuvenation and regeneration.* Escondido, CA: Bernard Jensen International.

Jensen, B. (1990). *A hunza trip with Dr. Bernard Jensen and the complete book of the wheel of health.* Escondido, CA: Bernard Jensen International.

Jensen, B. (1993). *Foods that heal: A guide tounderstanding and using thehealing powers of natural foods.* Wayne, NJ: Avery Publishing Group.

Kloss, J. (1971). *Back to Eden.* New York: Benedict Lust Publications.

Kunin, R. (1983). *Mega-nutrition for women.* New York: McGraw-Hill.

Kurtz, R., & Prestera, H. (1977). *Your body reveals.* New York: Bantam Books.

Lane, W. A., Sir. (1929). *The prevention of the diseases peculiar to civilization.* London: Faber & Faber.

Lappe, Frances Moore. (1976). *Diet for a Small Planet.* New York, New York. Ballantine.

Malstrom, S. (1980). *Own your own health.* New Canaan, CT: Keats Publishing.

McDougall, J. (1991). *The McDougall Program: 12 days to dynamic health.* New York: Penguin Books.

Pauling, L. (1970). *Vitamin C and the common cold.* San Francisco: W. H. Freeman & Company.

Pearson, D., & Shaw, S. (1982). *Life extension: A practical scientific approach.* New York: Warner Books.

Petrie, S. (1974). *Fat destroyer foods.* West Nyack, NY: Parker Publishing Company.

Rader, W. (1981). *Dr. Rader's no diet program for permanent weight loss.* Los Angeles: J. P. Tarcher.

Ratcliff, J. D. (1975). *I am Joe's body.* New York: Berkeley Books.

Restak, R. (1980). *The brain: The last frontier.* New York: Warner Books.

Robbins, J. (1987). *Diet for a new America.* Walpole, NH: Still Point Publishing.

Rosenthal, S. (1968). *Live high on low fat.* New York: J. B. Lippincott Co.

Shelton, H. (1978). *Fasting for renewal of life.* Chicago: Natural Hygiene Press.

Simmons, R. (1980). *Never say diet book.* New York: Warner Books.

Staff of the Bircher-Benner Clinic. (1973). *Bircher-Benner nutrition plan for skin problems* (Klaus Musmann, Trans.). Los Angeles: Nash Publishing.

Staff of the Bircher-Benner Clinic. (1977). *Bircher-Benner nutrition plan for liver and gallbladder problems* (Klaus Musmann, Trans.). New York: Pyramid Books.

Tarr, Y. Y. (1978). *The New York Times natural foods dieting book.* New York: Weathervane Books.

Trowbridge, J. P., & Walker, M. (1987). *The yeast syndrome.* New York: Bantam Books.

Wade, C. (1976). *The new enzyme catalyst diet.* West Nyack: Parker Publishing.

Walford, R. (1983). *Maximum life span.* New York: W. W. Norton & Company.

Walker, N. (1979). *Colon health: The key to a vibrant life.* Pheonix, AZ: O'Sullivan Woodside & Co.

Weil, A. (1988). *Health and healing: Understanding conventional and alternative medicine.* Boston: Houghton Mifflin.

Weil, A. (1995). *Spontaneous Healing.* New York: Fawcett Columbine.

Winick, M. (1982). *Growing up healthy: A parent's guide to good nutrition.* New York: William Morrow & Company.

About the Author

Dr. Kenneth Yasny is based in Los Angeles, where he has had a private practice in the field of nutrition for over 20 years. He studied educational psychology at California State College Northridge and received his Ph.D. in nutrition counseling from Ryokan College, where he also served as a professor and directed the Nutrition Program.

Dr. Yasny has acted as a consultant to Walt Disney Productions and various other corporations, as well as to many restaurants. He has lectured widely throughout the United States on nutrition, general health, weight control, and stress management.

Dr. Yasny is currently working on two new books and is updating has first book, *Talk To Me Body*.

The Colon Health Society

Hemorrhoids and constipation affect more than half of us living in the United States at some point in our lives, yet most of us are too embarrassed to talk about this problem. Information about hemorrhoids and constipation is not readily available, and what one can find is seldom helpful.

The Colon Health Society was formed to address these problems. We provide accurate, meaningful, and up-to-date information about causes, solutions, and lifestyle issues regarding hemorrhoids and constipation. We're particularly concerned about teaching people how to eliminate the pain and suffering that hemorrhoids and constipation often cause. We offer informative books, timely news reports, the best product information available anywhere, and special discounts to our members. Our approach is both medical and naturopathic.

Before you run out and purchase ointments, potions, or other remedies that probably won't work very well, contact us to find out what your choices really are and to decide what's best for you.

The products listed in this book and many other products relating to colon health are all available at a discount through the *Society*. Write to us, visit our website, or call our toll free number listed below.

The Colon Health Society
505 S. Beverly Drive #438
Beverly Hills, CA 90212
800-745-0791
*http://*www.colonhealth.com
esteem@starone.com

For information regarding this book, *The Colon Health Workbook,* "*The Colon Health Video,*" or boxed sets, please contact:

The Colon Health Society
505 S. Beverly Drive #438
Beverly Hills, CA 90212

Tel: 800-745-0791
Fax: 310-277-8952

www.colonhealth.com
esteem@starone.com